THE MULTIDISCIPLINARY PAIN CENTER

CURRENT MANAGEMENT OF PAIN

P. PRITHVI RAJ, SERIES EDITOR

The series, *Current Management of Pain*, is intended by the series editor and the publishers to provide up-to-date information on advances in the clinical management of acute and chronic pain and related research as quickly as possible. Both the series editor and the publishers felt that, although comprehensive texts are now available, they do not always cover the rapid advances in this field. Another format was needed to publish advances in basic sciences and clinical modalities and to bring them rapidly to the practitioners in the community. A questionnaire was sent to selected clinicians and, based on their responses, topics were chosen by the series editor. Editors of each volume were chosen for their expertise in the field and their ability to encourage other active pain specialists to contribute their knowledge.

PRINTED IN THE UNITED STATES.

Distributors

for the United States and Canada: Kluwer Academic Publishers, 101 Philip Drive, Assinippi Park, Norwell, MA 02061

for the UK and Ireland: Kluwer Academic Publishers, Falcon House, Queen Square, Lancaster LAl lRN, UK

for all other countries: Kluwer Academic Publishers Group, Distribution Centre, P.O. Box 322, 3300 AH Dordrecht, The Netherlands

Library of Congress Cataloging-in-Publication Data
The Multidisciplinary pain center: organization and personnel functions for pain management/edited by J.N. Ghia.
p. cm.—(Current management of pain; 1)
Includes index.
ISBN 0-89838-359-5
1. Intractable pain—Treatment. 2. Pain clinics. I. Ghia, J.N. (Jawahar N.), 1939–. II. Series.
[DNLM: 1. Outpatient Clinics, Hospital—organization & administration. 2. Pain—therapy. 3. Patient Care Team. WX 205 M961]
RB127. M84 1988
616. 047—dc19
DNLM/DLC
for Library of Congress
87-31389
CIP

THE MULTIDISCIPLINARY PAIN CENTER

ORGANIZATION AND PERSONNEL FUNCTIONS FOR PAIN MANAGEMENT

EDITED BY JAWAHAR N. GHIA

KLUWER ACADEMIC PUBLISHERS
BOSTON DORDRECHT LANCASTER

CONTENTS

CONTRIBUTING AUTHORS

Gerald M. Aronoff
Boston Pain Unit
Massachusetts Rehabilitation Hospital
125 Nashua Street
Boston, Massachusetts 02114

Steven F. Brena
Pain Control and Rehabilitation
Institute of Georgia, Inc.
350 Winn Way
Decatur, Georgia 30030

Benjamin L. Crue, Jr.
580 Oakcrest Drive
Durango, Colorado 81301

Jawahar N. Ghia
Anesthesia Pain Clinic
North Carolina Memorial Hospital
Chapel Hill, North Carolina 27514

John M. Gregg
Virginia Tech University and
Johns Hopkins University Medical Center
2727 South Main Street
Blacksburg, Virginia 24060

John D. Loeser
Department of Neurological Surgery
University of Washington
Seattle, Washington 98195

Patricia W. McAlary
Boston Pain Unit
Massachusetts Rehabilitation Hospital
125 Nashua Street
Boston, Massachusetts 02114

John C. Rowlingson
Pain Management Center
University of Virginia Medical Center
Box 293
Charlottesville, Virginia 22908

Timothy C. Toomey
Raleigh Pain Clinic
3410 Executive Drive
Suite 105
Raleigh, North Carolina 27609

Dennis C. Turk
Center for Pain Evaluation
and Treatment
c/o Eye and Ear Hospital, Pittsburgh
2302 Lothrop Street
Pittsburgh, Pennsylvania 15213

Sridhar V. Vasudevan
Department of Physical Medicine
and Rehabilitation
St. Joseph's Hospital
5000 W. Chambers Street
Milwaukee, Wisconsin 53210

SERIES EDITOR FOREWORD

The pain center/clinic is in the stage of transition. It has come a long way since chronic pain was a nonexistent entity and patients with difficult pain problems did not receive well-deserved attention or were lost in the busy practices of various specialty clinics. Thirty-five years ahead of the rest of us, John J. Bonica was the first physician who had a clear vision of a pain center's potential. Twenty years later, in response to loud public demands for relief of chronic pain, this idea was put into practice by a number of others on a somewhat larger scale. A team of specialists from various disciplines, trained in the management of chronic pain, now offer approaches ranging from simple outpatient care to inpatient hospitalization for comprehensive care including drug detoxification, behavior modification, and total rehabilitation of these patients. Hospitals have entered this arena with renewed enthusiasm. The pain center/clinic is now an established, accepted, and expanding method of providing care for chronic pain patients.

The chapters in this book are based on examples of multidisciplinary projects that deal comprehensively with management of chronic pain. Aimed primarily at the pain center/clinic in the university hospital setting, this book ranges from historical perspectives to current pain centers with their less orthodox methods of relieving chronic pain to the future of algology as a specialty. The book is indeed a broad spectrum in its coverage, with the chapters written by recognized and experienced pain authorities in their own specialty areas. These authors were chosen from various specialties to impart a true multidisciplinary flavor to this book.

So the time is ripe for Dr. Jawahar N. Ghia to tantalize us with a serious and thorough look at this subject. Dr. Ghia is a physician with the reputation and experience to explore these areas. He is a diplomate of the American Board of Anesthesiology and Director of Anesthesia Pain Clinic and Diagnostic and Therapeutic Block Services at the North Carolina Memorial Hospital in Chapel Hill, North Carolina. He has assembled a group of distinguished authorities, each with unique experience in the field, to pique the interest and intellect of all who wonder about the extent of the pain center's impact into what might be described as the "chronic pain market."

Surprisingly, there currently is no text that deals comprehensively and exclusively with pain clinics. This book is timely, readable, and helpful. It is one of the first books that discusses how to organize a pain center at a university hospital and is a worthy addition to the rapidly expanding bibliography of resources outlining the organization of the multidisciplinary pain clinic approach for management of chronic pain patients.

Dr Ghia's expertise in the field of the pain center comes from his first-hand experience in establishing the Multidisciplinary Pain Program at the University of North Carolina in 1972. In this book he gives much needed practical hints pertaining to the pain mechanism, diagnosis, and therapy of chronic pain syndromes, how to organize a pain center, and the problems inherent in establishing such a center. Dr. Ghia has presented a current and definitive picture of the pain center in a clear and concise manner valuable to anesthesiologists, surgeons, other physicians, hospital administrators, nurses, pain managers, students, residents, and those concerned with health planning and health economics.

P. Prithvi Raj

FOREWORD

The complaint of pain is one of the most common reasons for seeking health care. Although physicians usually manage acute pain successfully, there has been increasing evidence that the complaint of chronic pain is often a source of frustration for the physician and major disability for the patient. Indeed, society pays a very high price for chronic pain: in health care, wage replacement, disability payments, and loss of productivity. It has been estimated that chronic pain costs the United States over $66 billion per year.* Chronic pain is also an important cause of suffering, depression, marital stress, and unrealized human potential.

The medical issues surrounding chronic pain are themselves complex, but they do not suffice to explain the symptoms nor define the treatment of most chronic pain patients. During World War II, Dr. John Bonica perceived the need for a comprehensive evaluation of soldiers with complex pain complaints. He originated the idea of a multidisciplinary group of health care providers who would collectively evaluate the patient and make a comprehensive treatment recommendation. This group activity not only led to more accurate diagnosis and better treatment, but it provided the patient with an integrated treatment plan. In the traditional system of health care delivery, chronic pain patients tend to resemble billiard balls caroming off the side cushions as they wend their ways from doctor to doctor. In addition, some physicians and surgeons tend to blame the patient

* Bonica JJ: Past and current status of pain research and therapy. Sem Anesth vol V, no 2 (June), pp. 92–99, 1986.

for failure to respond to their treatments, as revealed by the all too common epithets of "psychosomatic pain" or "compensationitis." The multidisciplinary pain clinic asks the question, "Why does this patient complain of pain?" rather than blaming the patient for his illness.

In the mid-1960s a new dimension was added to the multidisciplinary pain clinic, based upon the work of Wilbert Fordyce at the University of Washington. He felt that the traditional, Cartesian model that dominated medical thinking was an inadequate explanation for the phenomena of chronic pain. He proposed a learning model stressing the role of environmental factors and an approach built upon both medical and behavioral analysis and treatment principles. From this powerful combination of medical and behavioral strategies grew new concepts such as the use of the pain cocktail to deal with iatrogenic polypharmacy, time-contingent rather than on-demand medications, progressive exercise programs built upon behavioral modification strategies, and behavioral shaping by controlled interactions with health care providers.

A few other pain clinics were launched in the early 1960s, and their contribution to our knowledge of chronic pain management must be recognized. It was, however, Bonica and Fordyce who stood at the forefront of this new movement. Health care delivery for chronic pain patients has undergone major changes in the past 15 years because of their efforts. National and international societies have been established, journals devoted to pain research and management are now numerous, and training programs that focus upon pain management are growing.

Not all factors in the development of the pain clinic have been beneficial to our society. The recognition that new health care strategies could be beneficial has led, in our free enterprise system, to the establishment of sham pain clinics, which do not offer appropriate diagnostic and therapeutic resources. Some pain clinics are nothing more than a single physician, psychologist, or alternative health care provider offering a single treatment modality for all patients. This has led to widespread confusion on the part of government agencies, third-party payers, and the public as to what is a good pain clinic and how to find one.

This book is an attempt to describe the development of multidisciplinary pain clinics and their present characteristics. It also looks ahead to the continued evolution of health care based upon multidisciplinary approaches. Each of the chapter authors has played a role in the development of the pain clinic movement and contributes knowledge and insights based upon personal experiences. This is, then, an "insider's" book, written by those who have done the work. It will help establish standards and goals for the next decade of continuing growth in this new type of health care delivery.

John D. Loeser

PREFACE

Increasingly, chronic pain patient care is becoming a multidisciplinary responsibility. Expertise in the fields of medical/surgical/psychiatric care has now increased to such an extent that no individual specialty can be expert in all aspects of chronic pain management. A greater understanding of pain mechanisms combined with improvement in psychiatric skill has allowed more and more success using rehabilitation of chronic pain patients with less and less use of invasive procedures. Organization of pain centers/clinics is the key to understanding chronic pain and the complex interrelationships between analgesic therapy, local anesthetic nerve blocks, psychiatric support, behavioral strategies, and the surgical regimens commonly used in treating chronic pain patients.

Since little has been written on the subject, it immediately poses the question, Why write a book? What is written in the literature is sparse, fragmentary, or distorted for dramatic effect and is not credible to the medical community and is contradictory or confusing to lay people.

Not a day goes by without some inquiry from physicians and community hospitals about how to organize a pain clinic. This book aims to provide all clinicians interested in the management of chronic pain patients with the specific information necessary to organize a center/clinic and to help them optimize the management of the individual patient, both in the university based hospital and the community setting. The book emphasizes the multidisciplinary pain team approach to patient management because it has been found superior to the traditional approach of nonintegrated individual therapies.

Publishers of the book requested that I use multiple authors. I wanted the anthology to read like a storybook written by one author rather than a series of choppy chapters with multiple authors. Therefore, I divided the book into seven chapters and sent an outline of each chapter to all authors, leaving enough flexibility for them to write what they wanted without impinging on each other. I wanted the authors to keep in touch with one another to synchronize their efforts and maintain continuity rather than becoming repetitious. Also, my general aim was to keep the story of the controversy as brief as possible. And that, in fact, is what I tried to do to the best of my ability. But, I must admit that the results have not been quite what I had expected. I have observed that each author has preconceived ideas or opinions, heroes to defend, and villains to punish. The authors defined and redefined chronic pain, took sides in approaches they used to diagnose and manage chronic pain, tried to establish themselves as pioneers in the field, or quarreled over credit.

In spite of the controversial nature of much that has been written, it is surprising how clearly the essential realities stand out if one takes the time to read all or most of the evidence. I am sure there are some errors in the book that no author writing on this subject can reasonably expect to avoid. However, it is my hope that my critics may not dwell exclusively upon them. We should grasp whatever opportunity this book affords to come to an agreement on essentials. Any work on a new and controversial subject is likely to invite stiff criticism, but I hope to be contributing to clarity rather than adding to confusion.

The contributors to this work have been chosen not only for their recognized knowledge and expertise in their field of pain management, but also because of their experience in providing such care to chronic pain patients. It is my hope that this effort will serve to make this type of care better understood, properly appreciated, more accessible, and more frequently utilized. The primary beneficiaries will be the patients so served. However, it is now well established that everyone who participates in management of chronic pain patients—pain managers, facilities involved, those responsible for payment for care, and the community at large—all benefit.

Acknowledgments

So many people have assisted me in the preparation of this book that it is impractical to try to name them all here. My appreciation begins with Dr. P. Prithvi Raj, who recommended me to be the editor of this book. It is obvious that this book could not have been written without the assistance of all contributing authors, who gave the quality to it. Many authors and publishers gave permission for their work to be quoted and reproduced, and due acknowledgment has been made in the text.

I thank Nancy Tripoli for editing the manuscripts of this book with diligence, always readily responding to the new demands of the editor, and Pat Stogner Bland, to whom I owe a special "thank you" for her editorial assistance and encouragement. Without the enthusiastic secretarial help of Tammy Hogan, Carol

Lloyd, and Ellen Stanford, it would not have been possible to start or finish this book. Many of the book's illustrations were prepared in the medical illustrations departments of the various authors' institutions. I am very grateful to Harold Rydberg for the excellent quality of figures provided by him for my chapters.

I now have the opportunity to acknowledge the departmental support and commitment to this project provided by Dr. Robert Vaughan, Professor and Chairman of the Department of Anesthesiology at the North Carolina Memorial Hospital. In recognition of my professional colleagues in the Department of Anesthesiology and the University of North Carolina Pain Program I wish to thank them for their assistance and the willingness of the staff to persevere because they believed this project to be worthwhile.

This book is dedicated to all my teachers and professional colleagues who helped establish the Multidisciplinary Pain Program at the University of North Carolina and inspired and stimulated me to learn: Kenneth Sugioka, M.D.; Edward Perl, M.D.; James P. Ferguson, M.D.; Stephen M. Mahaley, M.D.; John M. Gregg, Ph.D.. D.D.S; Timothy Toomey, Ph.D.; Ronald Woosley, M.D.; David Raft, M.D.; Philip Hirsch, Ph.D.; Raymond White, D.D.S; Timir Bannerjee, M.D.; Ernest Small, D.D.S., MS; and the late Gordon S. Dugger, M.D.

The list would not be complete without acknowledging the efforts of Barbara Ward and Jeffrey Stier of Kluwer Academic Publishers for their invaluable help in publishing this book. Finally, I wish to thank my wife, Dee, and our son, Gregory, and two daughters, Lisa and Audrey, who understood the trials and tribulations of writing a book and provided much needed moral support.

THE MULTIDISCIPLINARY PAIN CENTER

1. HISTORICAL PERSPECTIVES

BENJAMIN L. CRUE, JR.

Pain probably remains the most common symptom motivating humans to seek medical treatment. The complaint of pain and suffering extends back in time to the dawn of recorded history, from the Edwin Smith papyrus[1] to the story of Job in the Old Testament[2, 3]. Over the years, many remedies have been clinically successful to some degree, especially for acute pain due to injury or inflammation. This has been well documented by many authors, such as Keele[4] and Todd[5, 6]. Peripheral acting analgesics (aspirin from tree bark) and centrally acting narcotics (such as extract from the poppy) have been used for centuries.

Dentists, physicians, and anesthesiologists have long sought methods to relieve the often severe acute pain accompanying the surgeon's knife or dental extraction. Perhaps the modern history of scientific pain relief can be dated from the discovery and use of general anesthesia for the acute pain of surgery—nitrous oxide, chloroform, and ether.

The problem of etiology, mechanism, and effective therapy in chronic pain and suffering syndromes has, by comparison, often seemed mired in the historical past, in the realm of religion[7], mysticism, superstition, and mythology[8-11]. According to some recent references, such as the writings of Lewis[12], Yancey[13], Turner[14], and Kushner[15], we are not free from the moral judgment aspects of suffering. In fact, the root of the word *pain* is "punishment," rather than "alarm" or "warning."

BASIC PROBLEMS: ACUTE VERSUS CHRONIC PAIN

Simple as it first sounds, the problem of definitions and a taxonomy for classification of human pain states remains one of the major obstacles in the path of adequate communication, rational treatment conceptualizations, and further research in the suffering of mankind, both individually and collectively. There is still much disagreement, even among "experts" in the field.[16–26]

What is meant by the term *chronic pain*? Is it the same as acute pain that has gone on too long, or longer than can be explained by the initiating etiological factor? How the pejorative flavor does creep in!

Modern medicine has learned much in the last decade to explain and treat acute pain. By evaluating nociceptive input over the peripheral sensory nervous system and to the spinal cord and brain, usually due to injury and/or inflammation, much has been discovered about the peripheral and central neuroanatomy, neurophysiology, neurochemistry, and neuropharmacology of acute pain.

The study of peripheral prostaglandin metabolism led to better understanding of analgesia and development of many new pharmaceutical agents, such as non-steroidal anti-inflammatory drugs, which are clinically valuable to the rheumatologist, dentist, orthopedist, and sports medicine physician, among others. Concurrently, much has been learned about the centrally acting narcotics and the endorphins and enkephalins. The amount of research reported in this field staggers the imagination.[27] It has led to plausible explanations for the long-standing empirical clinical use of analgesic-narcotic combinations. We can anticipate the development of better agonists and antagonists and probably other pharmacological approaches still undreamed of. As a result, the modern physician can usually do an effective and intelligent job of treating clinical acute pain with nociceptive input.

The same cannot be said about chronic pain. For reasons sometimes difficult to fully elucidate, modern pain researchers and clinicians encounter a paradox in patients with chronic pain states. The newer agents, as well as the old standby analgesics and narcotic agents, often are not clinically effective, or at least not for very long. Yet many articles about modern pain treatment modalities that have proven effective in treating acute pain end with a statement or platitudinous prediction. The authors hope that newer or better agents will be found for chronic pain therapy by investigating the same line; that is, better modulation of the presumed underlying continued nociceptive input.

Chronic pain may not be just unusually long, ongoing acute pain. Perhaps it is time to question some of our underlying assumptions, conceptualizations, and beliefs.

PERIPHERALIST AND CENTRALIST CONCEPTS OF CHRONIC PAIN

A valuable distinction can be made between two presumptions about the etiology and treatment of chronic pain. Most physicians will find that both points of view have affected their past treatment of patients. The peripheralist versus centralist controversy concerning chronic pain[28–32] must be understood before considering evolution and present organization of pain clinics and centers[33].

Peripheralists interpret the phrase *chronic pain* to mean "enduring pain," no matter what its etiology. They believe that chronic pain can be viewed basically as a continuation of nociceptive input as in the acute pain medical model. When for some reason the original cause of the pain that initiated the nociceptive input continues longer than expected, or longer than usual, or even longer than seems reasonable, there is continuing pathophysiological change in the periphery at the site of the original injury, operation, or inflammation. Thus, peripheralists presume that there is continued peripheral input, not only in neuritis but in neuropathy and probably in neuralgia.[31] This is believed hypothetically possible because the peripheral pathology has not yet "healed correctly" or was not "fixed right" by the surgeon; or perhaps the continued nociceptive input originates in the inevitable scar. This reasoning ignores the observation that all patients have scarring after injury or surgery, yet most patients' pain decays and disappears.

Surprisingly, many psychologists appear to be peripheralists. This is the way we were all taught, and it appears to make good sense. Was not the original injury that started the pain syndrome located in the periphery, and does it not still hurt? Still, most experienced peripheralists admit that, with the passage of time, there is additional considerable psychological central " functional overlay." They do not claim that chronic pain is all due to peripheral nociceptive input.

Centralists interpret chronic pain to mean "pain that endures in the absence of enduring peripheral pathology." They believe that with any tissue damage and acute pain some kind of central "memory of pain" is established that can be hypothetically conceptualized as a "reverberating circuit," "internuncial pool," or "repetitive epileptiform firing" in the sensory neurons and networks of the central nervous system.[32] Under appropriate conditions the patient's brain can generate and continue to signal pain even further upward to the alarm bell in the patient's mind (which is referred to as the "conscious awareness of self" portion of central nervous system function). The pain can become chronic after a few days or several months.

After the etiological peripheral pathological condition heals, there is no need for (and no neurophysiological evidence of) the postulated continued peripheral nociceptive input. Centralists believe that such input then exists only in the imagination of the treating peripheralist physician. Thus neuralgia[31,34–46] becomes a third kind of pain, a central pain that is "referred" back to the periphery to that part of the body image from which the initial etiological nociceptive input occurred (often utilizing the mechanism of "memory").

In their psychoanalytic schematization of pain, Ramzy and Wallerstein labeled neuralgia, the centralists' term for chronic pain, as "neurotic bodily pain" and sandwiched it between peripheral or internal, also called somatic or visceral, nociceptive input acute pain (on the right) and mental, also called psychogenic or delusional, imaginary pain (on the left) (figure 1–1). The present author suggests that the term *neuralgic pain* is preferable because it presumes underlying uncontrolled epileptiform central firing mechanisms. He further suggests that while acute pain, with nociceptive input, was the triggering etiological agent, neuralgic

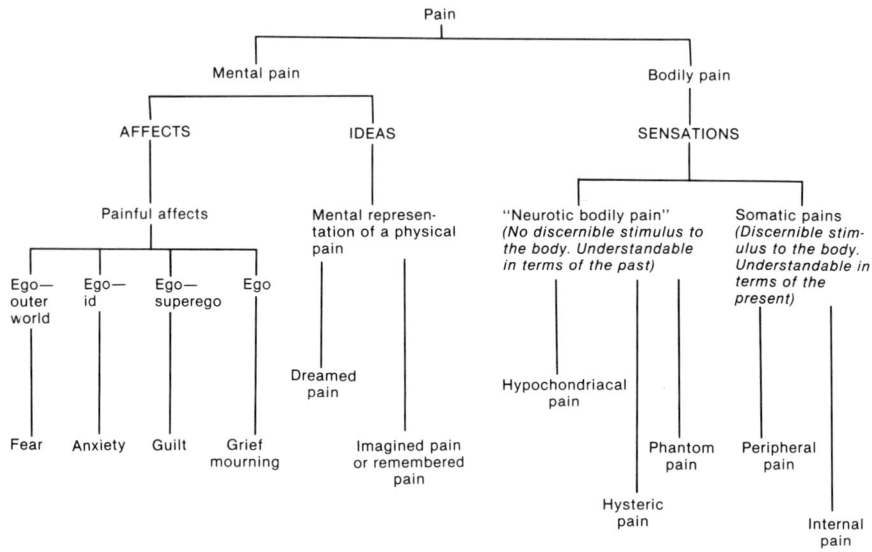

Figure 1–1. Psychoanalytic schematization of pain (Adapted from Ramzy and Wallerstein [47].)

pain becomes central psychosomatic pain and should be classed with hypochondriacal, hysterical, or phantom pain. According to the centralists' presumptions, *all* chronic pain is *always* psychosomatic, and pain not of this third type should not be labeled "chronic pain" no matter how long it has persisted clinically.

This taxonomy depends on a belief that in chronic pain, there is no longer any need to presume continued peripheral nociceptive input. Clinical experience has tended to demonstrate to many algologists that the chronic pain state stemming from continued peripheral nociceptive input is a widely held medical myth.[20]

Of course, both possible mechanisms exist and may be acting together in any one case of continued human suffering. The committed centralist would point out that were there any continued nociceptive input from the periphery, the pain should not be labeled chronic, no matter how long it has lasted clinically. The centralist would argue that the diagnosis of chronic pain should be reserved only for patients in whom there is presumably no longer any continued nociceptive afferent input from the periphery. This admittedly becomes a tautological classification, where "chronic" is equated with "central."

Table 1–1 contains the author's classification of pain. An attempt to place patients in these categories, though not always possible, will help to clarify treatment strategies. Some patients, without question, have chronic underlying organic pathophysiological conditions, or disease entities, such as rheumatoid arthritis (with recurrent flare-up of acute joint pain) or chronic osteoarthritis where, with certain movement, the spurs on the spine may irritate nerve roots and give

Table 1–1. Temporal classification of pain complaints

1. Acute: up to a few days in duration, mild or severe with cause known or unknown, presumed nociceptive input (the "fix me" medical model).
2. Subacute: few days to a few months in duration (though no longer an emergency, in most ways treated like acute pain).
3. Recurrent acute: recurrent or continued nociceptive input from underlying chronic pathological process, that is, arthritis (either rheumatoid or osteoarthritis).
4. Ongoing acute: due to uncontrolled malignant neoplastic disease, with continued nociceptive input.
5. Chronic: benign, nonneoplastic, usually more than six months, no known nociceptive peripheral input, but pain often made more severe by any type of subsequent sensory input; basically a "central" pain, but with seemingly adequate coping by the patient.
6. Chronic intractable benign pain syndrome (CIBPS): chronic pain with poor patient coping; pain becomes central focus of the patient's existence (no known nociceptive peripheral input).

recurrent pain. Although these patients have chronic pathology, their pain would be classified recurrent acute pain, with recurrent nociceptive input—category 3 of table 1–1. There are many entrapment syndromes, not just median nerve carpal tunnel disorders, but extruded discs with compressed nerve roots, in which the author is ready to undertake a surgical approach after adequate conservative therapy has been tried. They also fall in category 3 of table 1–1. Other category 3 specific pain syndromes in which operative intervention is indicated include major causalgia with a partial lesion to a mixed motor sensory nerve, for which repetitive sympathetic nerve blocks (and occasionally sympathectomy) are definitely indicated—and when done promptly the results are excellent. In primary trigeminal neuralgia or tic douloureux, when anticonvulsants have failed (or the patient has proved allergic to Tegretol, Dilantin, or Baclofen), any one of a number of neurosurgical procedures may be efficacious and definitely indicated.

Continued nociceptive input from advancing pathology, such as malignancy (which is the only cause of such ongoing nociceptive input), would fall in category 4. Both nerve blocks and neurosurgical operative intervention have a large role to play in helping the unfortunate patients in category 4.

Categories 5 and 6 are reserved for chronic pain patients in whom, by definition, there is no longer any nociceptive input. We have little epidemiological knowledge about patients in category 5, who are coping and do not seek medical care. Patients in category 6 have continuing suffering but no continued nociceptive input. An underlying central generator mechanism causes the chronic pain. They have developed poor adaption, with poor coping skills. Chronic pain now forms the center of their existence. In this category are found the chronic pain patients with full-blown chronic intractable benign pain syndrome (CIBPS), which has been defined repeatedly by authors such as Pinsky. Table 1–2 is from his description of chronic pain with general characteristics and the epiphenomena that accompany this syndrome.[48-52]

What predisposing factors lead to the establishment of such a central generator mechanism? Table 1–3 suggests that both organic and functional environmental factors may predispose to central pain states. Every neurosurgeon who sees

Table 1–2. Chronic intractable benign pain syndrome (CIBPS)

General characteristics of pain

1. Cannot be shown to be causally related to the here-and-now with any active pathophysiologic or pathoanatomic process.
2. Has an antecedent history of generally ineffective medical and surgical intervention in the pain problem.
3. Has come to be accompanied by disturbed psychosocial function that includes the pain complaint and the epiphenomena that accompany it.

Epiphenomena

1. Substance use disorders of varying severity with their attendant CNS side effects.
2. Multiple surgical procedures or pharmacologic treatments with their own morbid side effects separate from those related to above.
3. Escalated decrease in physical functioning related to accompanying pain and/or fear that this pain is a signal of increased bodily harm and damage.
4. Escalated hopelessness and helplessness as persistent or increased dysphoria does not give way in the face of mounting numbers of "newer" or different treatment interventions.
5. Emotional conflicts with medical care delivery personnel (doctors, nurses, therapists, technicians), which result in therapeutic goal interference.
6. Interpersonal emotional conflicts with significant others.
7. Lasting, unpleasant mood and affect changes.
8. Decrease in feelings of self-esteem, self-worth, and self-confidence.
9. Escalated withdrawal and loss of gratification from psychosocial activity.
10. Decreased ability to obtain pleasure from the life process, reflected in the presence of profound demoralization and, at times, significant depression.

Table 1–3. Predisposing central factors to chronic pain

1. Organic lesion with CNS
   (a) Pathological (example: poststroke).
   (b) Physiological from abnormal peripheral input (example: causalgia).
   (c) Mixture of pathological and physiological (possible example: tic douloureux).
2. Possible "genetic" inherited defects or, at least, individual differences.
3. "Functional" environmental factors from physiologically normal but psychologically often "abnormal" peripheral input from external milieu.
   (a) Past input into memory storage including early nurturance ("psychosomatic").
   (b) Reactive factors to acute pain (as often the etiological trigger) ("somatopsychic").
   (c) Mixture of the two (the CIBPS syndrome).

patients with poststroke pain, pain in multiple sclerosis, trigeminal neuralgia, causalgia, or any of the deafferentation hypersensitivity syndromes often resulting in reflex sympathetic dystrophy, is well aware that many central pain states are "more organic" than other psychosomatic chronic pain syndromes.

The major problem with the classification system in table 1–1 is disagreement between therapeutic personnel about which patients should be placed in category 6. The centralist believes that most patients with continuing suffering belong in category 6 and that these patients, in whom there is no longer any nociceptive peripheral input to block or to fix, represent a large group. Patients in this group experienced many of the past failures of anesthesiological nerve blocks and neurosurgical chordotomies, after the initial beneficial placebo response had worn off. These are also the patients who are costing Americans at least $90 billion a year in lost wages, costly medical care, third-party payments, or disability awards in litigation settlements for pain and suffering.[59]

Peripheralists will conversely state that category 6 is a small group of patients, in whom the centrally generated pain is all psychogenic. This small percentage of all pain patients, along with patients in categories 3 and 4, they would label as having chronic pain syndromes. The individual neurosurgeon must decide whether the individual patient with the continuing complaint of pain fits into category 3, which warrants further attempt at decreasing presumed continued nociceptive input, or into category 6, for which treatment, by definition, is going to be inherently psychological or psychiatric. Thus, physicians may not object to a classification system that labels chronic pain as psychosomatic, provided that they are individually free to put in category 3 a patient who has had "real" organic peripheral pathology. They can then presume underlying continuing pathophysiology and continued nociceptive input, which they are also presumably trained to treat, accompanied by some percentage of centrally generated psychological "functional overlay".[29]

Neurosurgeons have a tremendous repertoire of surgical procedures aimed at pain relief[53]. However, it is time for neurosurgeons and those who rely on nerve block therapy to admit that some chronic pain patients, as outlined in category 6, cannot benefit from such procedures. Anesthesiological peripheral nerve blocks as well as neurosurgical rhizotomies, chordotomies, and tractotomies have not worked in a sufficient percentage of such patients followed postoperatively over an adequate course of time and can no longer be considered acceptable treatments. This conclusion is reached with considerable sadness, not only because the writer is a neurosurgeon, but because experience has shown that this statement may be misunderstood. In no way does it imply that patients with organic pathology and nociceptive input, whom we would put in category 3 as having recurrent acute pain, should not receive neurosurgical attention.

These statements about chronic pain lead to the generalization that nerve blocks and neurosurgical procedures are not indicated in patients with chronic pain syndromes in the absence of a nociceptive component. It has been the poor results from all forms of treatment of such patients, including peripheral and epidural nerve blocks, and often multiple mutilating neurosurgical interventions, that have been the impetus for the development of pain clinics and multidisciplinary pain centers.

EVOLUTION OF PAIN CLINICS AND PAIN CENTERS

Over the last two decades there has been a development in the field of pain treatment that should be of interest to all. This is the development of the specialized pain clinic and pain center. Although the impetus was demonstrated failure of current medical and surgical treatment of chronic pain patients, there was also a concomitant belief that the alternative of therapy at a pain center by a multidisciplinary trained pain team might have something additional to offer. Many multidisciplinary (and later interdisciplinary) pain teams evolved when outpatient pain clinics found themselves failing in their missions and pain clinic directors became dissatisfied with their inability to help many chronic pain syndrome patients.

The term *pain clinic* here means a specialized facility that treats patients with chronic pain on an outpatient basis. The word *clinic* means outpatient care, rather than free care (as was once true in England and in many parts of the United States.) As these pain teams were assembled they evolved in many different directions. Often nonmedical team members were added, and the term *interdisciplinary*[54] is appropriate. These teams often included physical therapists and occupational therapists for the reconditioning of the chronic pain patient's body, which had atrophied through disuse. They may have included a psychologist, or more rarely a psychiatrist, for the treatment of the recognized central or functional aspects of the chronic pain complaints. The development usually mirrored the beliefs, training, and specialty of the original pain clinic directors, as well as the referral patterns and the needs of the individual host institution. The pain clinic may have evolved into a pain center in a cancer hospital, in a university or general hospital setting, or in an orthopedic, rheumatological, or dental service. As more and more physicians were assembled, first as consultants and then as members of pain teams, the programs became multidisciplinary.

When inpatient services were added, the pain clinics became known as "pain centers" and often became comprehensive, interdisciplinary, multidisciplinary, interdepartmental pain centers, although the number of institutions that could truly be called comprehensive pain centers has remained relatively small.

The author suggested[55] that a pain center should include (1) an outpatient pain clinic for triage, diagnosis, and treatment; (2) an inpatient pain service, of whatever specialty (e.g., neurology, neurosurgery, orthopedics, rheumatology), for those patients who could not be treated optimally for their pain on an outpatient basis; and (3) a specialized pain unit for both inpatient and outpatient treatment of conditions believed to be largely psychosomatic (in category 6 of table 1–1), where psychiatry and psychology was in charge. It was our belief then, and is an even stronger belief today, that treatment here is best centered on group psychotherapy. It was also believed that in a developing field, in addition to the three components listed, a comprehensive pain center should include (4) facilities for clinical and basic research, and (5) a component for teaching, either through a medical school affiliation or by having approved pain fellowships in this new field of chronic pain treatment, which has since come to be known as the specialty of algology.

Though there had been symptom- or syndrome-oriented clinics specializing in headache and lower back problems—even an attempt in Texas during World War II to start a true team approach to the treatment of pain for members of the armed services—the present concept of the comprehensive pain center appears to be an outgrowth of two prototype pain clinics started in 1960 that evolved into comprehensive, multidisciplinary pain centers over the years. The author founded a pain clinic, affiliated with the University of Southern California School of Medicine, at the City of Hope in Duarte, that continued for 21 years (1960–1980). This pain team, now known as the New Hope Pain Center, was moved in 1980 to Alhambra, California, and then in 1984 to Pasadena. Dr. John Bonica[56], at the University of Washington in Seattle, also started a pain clinic in 1960, which has also evolved into a comprehensive pain center. There has been a marked contrast between the two, however, in that the University of Washington Pain Center[57–61] evolved out of a peripheralist-oriented nerve block clinic run by an anesthesiologist (with the association of psychologist Dr. W.E. Fordyce), whereas the New Hope Pain Center evolved along centralist lines (when this neurosurgeon called psychiatrist Dr. J.J. Pinsky for help with chronic pain patients).

While this movement appears to have started about 1960, there may well be other centers, unknown to the author, that preceded these. Other inpatient pain treatment centers were soon started in the United States: in Minneapolis, with Donlin Long; Atlanta, with Steven Brena; Portland, with Joel Seres and Richard Newman; Boston, with Nate Hollister and Gerald Aronoff; and, Boulder, with Richard Stieg. It appears that the concept caught on rather slowly. In 1976, *Medical World News* reported on 17 pain centers in the United States; in 1977, the American Society of Anesthesiologists published a directory listing 243 pain clinics and pain centers in the United States. An updated issue in 1979 listed 277 clinics and centers; but many pain clinics and centers were omitted and the listings included only self-evaluations. At present it is estimated that there are more than 1,000 pain clinics and pain centers in the United States (more than 60 of them in southern California alone).

Unfortunately, while a real need resulted in pain teams at developing pain centers, and treatment by well-organized pain teams has been medically worthwhile for patients with chronic pain syndromes[51,62–65] and cost[66] effective (including patients with on-the-job injuries), there has recently been such a rush to get into this field that the author believes there is the danger of a backlash. The difficulty is compounded by the fact that there have been no truly acceptable prospective or double-blind studies to demonstrate proof of medical effectiveness. There are as yet no adequate guidelines for evaluating pain clinics and pain centers, to inform either referring physicians or the public about their proven competence. Stieg and Williams'[66] attempts to show cost effectiveness are estimates, and all may not agree with all aspects of their formula. However, they did point out the impressive figure of a quarter of a million dollars as the cost for each compensation-covered male with a back injury on the job who was lost to permanent disability.

Several factors have caused this recent acceleration of pain center development. With the tightening of hospital admission guidelines, and the establishment of utilization committees, PSROs, and HSAs, some areas of the country (such as southern California) have too many hospital acute-care medical/surgical beds. A number of hospital administrators have found that pain unit beds are inexpensive to operate, and there often has been considerable impetus to find someone (even if not a physician) to act as a pain program director, often at least nominally under the auspices of a medical director. Pain treatment programs (as well as alcohol rehabilitation programs) have sometimes been started for less than altruistic reasons. Furthermore, there has been considerable recent public education on pain problems through the media, perhaps starting with acupuncture following President Nixon's trip to China. This has accelerated the interest in pain treatment by many modality-specific therapies (everything from acupuncture to transcutaneous electrical stimulation to biofeedback to hypnosis). A number of pain clinics are marginally supervised and often unimodal and nothing more than outpatient treatment offices run primarily for financial gain. Along with this has been an impetus to start more outpatient specialty pain clinics to treat specific syndromes—headache clinics, lower back clinics, rheumatology pain clinics, sports medicine clinics, and other similar programs. Every hospital now wants its own pain therapy programs, as do many smaller cities. Inpatient services in comprehensive pain centers can now be found in acute-care hospital settings, in rehabilitation facilities, and in psychiatric institutions. However, because of recent cost containment efforts, many pain centers are now focusing more on outpatient clinic treatment whenever possible.

In an attempt to answer a demonstrated need, both for the public as well as for the medical profession, and with the urging of some third-party payers such as major insurance companies, an effort was made, starting in 1978, to establish guidelines or criteria for pain clinics and pain centers through the American Pain Society, which now has some 800 members (about half of whom are physicians) and which is a national chapter of the International Association for the Study of Pain. Considerable discussion ensued, and, with many different medical specialties involved (as well as psychologists, dentists, physical therapists, nurses, and basic researchers), it proved to be a very formidable task to reach a consensus. Finally in 1981 the surveying and certification agency of Tucson, known as CARF (Commission on Accreditation of Rehabilitation Facilities), which had already been surveying and accrediting rehabilitation facilities for some 14 years, announced that its board of directors had decided to accept the task of both setting up criteria and surveying pain clinics and pain centers in the United States, on a voluntary request basis. At their request, 13 algologists with experience in treating chronic pain patients met in Chicago in July 1982, and tentative criteria for minimum standards for a CARF survey mechanism for both outpatient pain clinics and inpatient comprehensive pain centers, were agreed upon. These were submitted first to the American Pain Society, and changes were made by the board of directors at the annual meeting of the American Pain Society in Miami in October 1982. These amended criteria were then accepted and approved by the board of directors of CARF, and surveying of pain clinics and pain centers (as to their actually meeting the agreed-upon criteria) was begun in July 1983. These initial minimal criteria should be of interest. (They can be obtained by writing CARF at 2500 North Pantano Road, Tucson, AZ 85715.) To date, some

59 pain centers and outpatient pain clinics have been certified.

In the spring of 1987, the author will again be joining a second CARF-sponsored national advisory committee in Chicago (four years after the first such meeting) to review present standards and criteria for pain clinics (outpatient) and pain centers (inpatient) to see if updating is advisable. We will also be considering standards and criteria for cancer pain treatment centers, as well as syndrome-oriented pain clinics (headache, backache, and so on). There are no immediate plans to tackle the problem of monomodality pain treatment clinics (such as physiotherapists and neurologists using TENS units; acupuncture and hypnotherapy parlors; or even anesthesiologists' nerve block clinics). An eclectic[67] approach is certainly necessary!

Recently, several neurosurgeons have expressed concern about the appropriateness of nonneurosurgeons participating in a team decision regarding whether neurosurgeons should, in any specific patient, implant either spinal or deep brain stimulating electrodes or perform a stereotactic prefrontal lobotomy, cingulotomy, or other such procedure. There has been more communication to the author (especially from his fellow neurosurgeons) along these lines than there has been the expected outcry from operators of proliferating outpatient pain clinics using only such measures as nerve blocks, hypnosis, acupuncture, transcutaneous electrical nerve stimulation units, and biofeedback. It must be pointed out that this CARF survey is entirely voluntary at present, and it is designed for inpatient and outpatient chronic pain management programs—not for neurosurgical or anesthesiological services in university centers that may be treating patients with pain complaints as part of their regular programs.

It is hoped, however (at least by the author), that if and when CARF certification has become established, two factors may begin to play a role: (1) As more institutions request voluntary certification as having met the minimal criteria, the standards can be appropriately tightened, where and when indicated, by the established process as formulated by the CARF organization, and (2) as insurance carriers, legislators, and the public in general become aware of CARF certification, certification may become a prerequisite of third-party payment (and thus we can envision an economic force utilized for improvement of patient care). This requirement has recently been passed into law in Florida, thanks to the efforts of Shams and other algologists. Similar regulations are now being considered in Maryland and Washington. Not everyone may agree with the author's opinion as to the desirability of these hoped-for changes, but they now appear inevitable.

Comprehensive pain centers, when they are adequately directed, staffed, and operated, do have much to offer the practicing clinician, and have demonstrated a better approach to the treatment of CIBPS patients, whose condition is basically psychosomatic (category 6 in table 1–1). Such centers offer a referral resource for all those truly interested in helping their patients with chronic pain.

Furthermore, such pain teams offer an alternative method of treating pain in cancer patients and in those dying of cancer within the hospice concept. (An en-

Table 1–4. Three major components of the suffering process in patients with pain from cancer

1. Continued nociceptive input.
2. Central psychological mechanisms, as in CIBPS.
3. Threat of impending death from the cancer.

tire new chapter would be needed to do justice to the history of the benefit from the hospice movement.) Too many cancer patients are having their medical treatment needs met by the new specialty of medical oncology (largely with newer chemotherapeutic agents for attacking the neoplasm) only to have their ongoing suffering receive too little recognition and therapy.

Many terminal cancer patients can be relieved without nerve blocks or mutilating neurosurgical procedures (even if they can now often be done percutaneously)[68,69] by the judicious use of a cancer pain team trained in the use of psychological support, utilizing the family maximally, and by education of the patient in the use of antidepressants and oral narcotics[70,71]. Cancer center algologists such as Foley in New York and T. Brechner in Los Angeles should be considered within the fold of pain center clinicians. Table 1–4 reminds us that the patient with cancer pain is not just having continued ongoing nociceptive input pain, to be blocked by the anesthesiologist or more permanently interrupted by the neurosurgeon. Such a patient is a human being capable of reacting emotionally with all the same or similar unconscious psychological defense mechanisms as is the CIBPS patient. Furthermore, in the terminal cancer pain patient, the ever present threat of impending death adds an intensity and an immediacy usually not seen in the CIBPS patient.

Patients without cancer but with continued nociceptive input and recurrent acute pain from underlying chronic disease entities, such as rheumatoid arthritis, can often benefit from the support offered by an affiliated pain center with a trained pain therapy team.

The psychologists and psychiatrists on an experienced pain treatment team also can help in the preoperative evaluation of selected neurosurgical operative candidates. Even patients with extreme anxiety can develop operative conditions accompanied by the complaint of pain. The preoperative and postoperative patient can often be helped by support from an experienced pain therapy team, and that support must be experienced to be really appreciated, both by the patient and by the surgeon. Preoperative evaluation does have predictive value, and chronic pain syndrome patients can often be helped and supported during subsequent intercurrent problems with acute nociceptive input pain.

In assessing results of therapy in pain clinics and pain centers, five factors must always be kept in mind (table 1–5).[71] This is true both for patients with cancer pain and those with CIBPS. Time will not be taken to discuss this further in detail. But, before discussing modalities of therapy and immediate results for chronic pain, the classification problem must first be solved so that we are not comparing apples to oranges. A patient with CIBPS cannot be compared to an

Table 1–5. Factors to be taken into account in considering results of therapeutic modalities in chronic or cancer pain

1. Patient selection
2. Goals of therapy
3. Specific modalities of treatment
4. Immediate results
5. Long-term results and recidivism rates

arthritic patient with recurrent acute pain. Futhermore, in chronic pain therapy, because of the sometime profound and long-lasting placebo effect (that each treating physician is loathe to recognize and admit), short-range results mean almost nothing. Many surgical patients are relieved of their pain at the time of postoperative hospital discharge, only later to hurt again; again surgeons are reluctant to study and admit their long-range recidivism rates. Only long-term results are of much value in patients treated for chronic pain. Who knows, some of the CIBPS patients with poor short-term results from pain clinic therapy even get better after they return home!

We cannot conclude this introductory chapter without commenting on two important but negative and seemingly long-range trends that appear to be impinging on the formation and recognition of pain clinics and centers, and indeed on the entire algology movement: (1) socioeconomic factors and (2) psychological resistance to the use of psychology and/or psychiatry in chronic pain patients. These issues are difficult to discuss separately, as the subjects become intertwined, as once again the taxonomy problem further confuses the muddle.

First, a few disjointed comments about some socioeconomic factors. When starting the pain center at City of Hope in 1960 we had little problem in getting full payment for eight or more weeks of inpatient therapy for chronic pain patients. In the early seventies Pinsky worked with psychiatrist Ron Mintz, head of rehabilitation reimbursement for Blue Cross of southern California, our Medicare intermediary. A Medicare bulletin resulted, which gave 80 percent payment for up to eight weeks for Medicare patients in our inpatient pain center. Since our patients were largely female, average age in the mid-fifties, who had been disabled by pain on an average for seven years, the majority of chronic pain patients in those early years were totally disabled and under Social Security and covered by Medicare. Thus, Medicare patients really enabled us to build, initially at this small charitable cancer hospital, a full-time pain team of ten members at the doctorate level—seven physicians and three Ph.D.s. The physicians were two neurosurgeons, two neurologists, one psychiatrist, one anesthesiologist, and one orthopedist and rehabilitation physiatrist, along with two psychologists and a neurophysiologist. This already multi-and interdisciplinary team was expanded to 20 with the inclusion of a full or part-time physical therapist, occupational therapist, recreational therapist, movement and art therapist, pain unit nurse, cancer pain team nurse, vocational rehab counselor, social worker, pharmacist, and dietician.

In those heady days we were exhilarated by what we were learning about chronic pain states and by certain good results. Dr. Bonica at Seattle had likewise built a well-known and distinguished pain team at the University of Washington. Both teams were often referred to as "Cadillac" models by visiting pain treaters eager to start their own pain clinics and pain centers.

As the number of pain treatment centers grew, the inevitable (in hindsight) happened. Medicare cut reimbursement to six weeks, then to four weeks. Then with the advent of PSROs the need to hospitalize chronic pain patients was challenged—both in acute med/surg beds, or psych beds, or even rehab beds. After 1983 we were not paid for inpatient therapy by Medicare. Helen Neal[72] was correct when she described a "Politics of Pain." While she referred mainly to the peripheralist-oriented pain center at the University of Washington, she quite succinctly pointed out in 1978 that before World War II the majority of patients had acute disease but that now 80 percent of patients have a chronic illness. There is not enough money to give anywhere near optimum care to the patient needing management rather than cure for chronic syndromes such as chronic pain. With the advent of Medicaid (MediCal in California) the difference among states became important. MediCal never paid for the treatment of chronic pain patients, as Medicaid did in Massachusetts.

One of the bright spots was the recognition by comprehensive insurance carriers in a few states of the value of pain clinic therapy to their injured workers—usually younger and, most often, male. This benefit was valued in spite of the obvious problem of secondary gain related to on-the-job injury and probable subsequent litigation. However, carriers usually insisted on outpatient pain clinic therapy and limited treatment for three or four weeks. A number of outpatient clinics did well, attracting a large number of these injured workers (e.g., Seres and Newman in Portland, Brena and Chapman in Atlanta, and Stieg in Boulder).

Nevertheless, the shift from inpatient to outpatient therapy often eliminated treatment for chronic pain patients with private insurance—their insurance most often only covered in-hospital therapy. When insurance industry leaders (as well as large HMO and union and industry leaders) were approached, they uniformly recommended that algologists stimulate "consumer demand." This is an undertaking that both the many chronic pain patients (with their pain state and almost uniformly poor self-image) and the nation's few algologists have appeared ill-equipped to undertake. This will be a massive mission—despite the fact that Helen Neal points out that a few dedicated laymen *can* make a difference.

One example of the difficulty can be illustrated by the actions of Blue Shield of California and California Physicians Service (the physicians' own company). (To this day the Blue Shield Medical Policy Committee in California "sets the tone" for Blue Cross and for much of the rest of the nation as well.) The director (a former practicing physician) refused to allow payment for pain centers and pain clinics because they were not demonstrably "medically effective." After several algologists testified at subsequent hearings, this ruling was reversed; many compliments were heard, with the admonition to keep up the good work. But the director still denied payment because we had "not proven" that pain clinics were "cost effective." After several more meetings it was pointed out that although we believed pain clinics were cost effective, such proof required financial information to which physicians were not privy but Blue Shield was. (Several requests to undertake a joint pilot study were ignored.) To expect algologists to prove cost effectiveness of pain clinic treatment thus seemed unfair. Coronary bypass surgery had just been approved for financial reimbursement—with little testimony demonstrating long-range medical benefit and none at all related to cost effectiveness. Not even appendectomy had never been so questioned! The director of Blue Shield reluctantly agreed, but then made another startling discovery: *All* pain treatment was "rehabilitation," even if carried out in acute med surg beds or in a psychiatric institution. And, surprisingly, Blue Shield contracts did not provide for rehabilitation services, nor were they likely to do so. The financial exposure for treating chronic illnesses—and chronic pain was so included—was likened to "opening Pandora's box"!

Attempts to cut costs by changing from an inpatient to an outpatient mode (which reduced costs almost one-half, by eliminating the hospital) led to an even smaller pool of potential chronic pain patients and excluded many with private hospital insurance, which had heretofore been considered adequate coverage. At the same time, the number of medical centers wanting a pain treatment team was increasing.

One consequence of the further tightening of economic purse strings under the present federal administrators (as well as Gramm-Rudman) has been the inevitable downgrading of newer pain teams. They are now often composed of treaters with fewer years of training and are no longer truly multidisciplinary with several physicians in the "Cadillac" model. The team leader is often a nonphysician (e.g., a psychologist, nurse, physical therapist,) entitled a "program director." The one physician is often a part-time "medical director" who uses other physicians as consultants on an as-needed basis. The psychotherapists are often master's degree level, with a part-time Ph.D. psychologist as supervisor. Under such circumstances, the CARF survey and accreditation is certainly needed to prevent abuse by part-time medical directors to prevent their becoming physician prostitutes, signing prescriptions one afternoon a week on the way to the golf course!

The situation also enables such "downgraded" pain teams to include other less formally trained members, including lay volunteers, former pain patients, nutritionists, acupuncturists, hypnotists, biofeedback technicians, massage specialists, swimming instructors, exercise and movement therapists. Thus, attempts to cut costs, as well as the resistance of many patients and medical directors to the use of psychiatry and psychology (to be discussed in the following paragraphs), have given impetus to the holistic movement. While the holistic approach may well have merit, as pointed out by Frank[73], the exclusion of psychiatry and the inclusion of the occult by some pain clinics certainly must make the traditionally trained physician wonder whether fringe elements have indeed taken over the chronic pain treatment field[74].

Any historical review of the algology movement and the development of pain clinics and centers[75–77] would be incomplete without a discussion of "resistance." This concept is long familiar to psychiatry. If one now approaches chronic pain patients from the centralist's viewpoint (that all chronic pain is always all psychosomatic), it is no wonder that patient resistance will be fierce! But resistance can be overcome.[64] And the patient's family can be won over. All are initially convinced upon entering the pain team therapy program that they still have something wrong, out there where the pain is, and where they were injured or operated. They are fixed in the acute pain model.

Patient resistance pales into insignificance, however, when compared to the intransigence of many of our physician colleagues. The inability of the medical profession to accept psychotherapy in the treatment of chronic pain, let alone the centralists' psychosomatic chronic pain concept[78], can result in confusion and inadequate or incorrect therapy for the chronic pain patient. For example, take the recent AMA guide[79] for impairment rating (that naturally affects the disability rating). The AMA Permanent Impairment Guide, on page 73, discusses pain and peripheral nerves; "Pain may be defined as a unique complex made up of afferent stimuli interacting with the emotional or affective state of the individual, and modified by that individual's past experience and present state of mind. The two constituents, neural stimulation and central reaction, are extremely variable in make-up and duration." The peripheralist bias on continued nociceptive input (in the here and now) shows through, with no allowance for pain originating with injury and acute pain but is now all psychosomatic (central pain) when it becomes chronic. The Impairment Guide further states: "Complaints of pain that cannot be substantiated as above are not considered within the scope of this chapter." Also, apparently, not within the scope of physical impairment, as pain is not considered further anywhere else in this recent official AMA manual, this is apparently left at the end of the guide manual to the psychiatrist under the section on mental and behavioral disorders, and to the D.S.M. III under the apparent belief all other pain must be "psychogenic." For a discussion of the problems in relating chronic pain to the D.S.M. III refer to Aronoff[65] and Morse[67].

Thus, sadly (to the author) the future of algology is still in doubt. The pain team (and the pain center and pain clinic) movement, which has proven medically effective in many patients with chronic pain, when all else has failed, may not be viable in our present socioeconomic climate, especially with so much individual patient and collective medical resistance still to be overcome.

It will be of interest to see how such a chapter on historical perspectives concerning pain clinics will read in the next century. Psychotherapy is still suspect[80], but it is the best we have presently for understanding and treating chronic pain.

REFERENCES

1. Breasted JH (ed): The Edwin Smith Surgical Papyrus. Chicago: University of Chicago Press, 1930, p 135.
2. Job. Book of Holy Bible, King James Version.
3. Bakan D: Disease, Pain, and Sacrifice—Toward a Psychology of Suffering. Boston: Beacon Press, 1968.
4. Keele KD: Anatomies of Pain. Springfield, Ill: Charles C Thomas, 1957.
5. Todd E: Pain: Historical perspectives. In: Crue BL (ed) Chronic Pain. New York: Spectrum, 1979.
6. Todd E: Origins of modern psychiatry in the sixteenth century witchcraze. In: Reflections Through a Murky Crystal. Pasadena, Calif., 1986.
7. Brena SF: Pain and Religion, a Psychophysiological Study. Springfield, Ill: Charles C Thomas, 1972.
8. MacKay C: Extraordinary Popular Delusions and the Madness of Crowds. London: Moonday Press, 1841.
9. Hilton J: Rest and Pain. London: G. Bill and Sons, 1863.
10. Die Schmerzphanomene Bei Inneren Krankheiten irhe Pathogenese and Differentialdiagnose. Wein und Leipzig, 1906.
11. Bulfinch T: Mythology. Fuller E (ed) New York: Dell Publishing, 1959.
12. Lewis CS: The Problem of Pain. New York: Macmillan, 1962.
13. Yancey P: Where Is God When It Hurts? Grand Rapids: Loudervan, 1977.
14. Turner D: Care in evil. In: Commitment to Care. Old Greenwich, Conn.: Devin-Adair, 1978.
15. Kushner HS: When Bad Things Happen to Good People. New York: Shocken Books, 1981.
New York: Shocken Books, 1981.
16. Crue BL, Carregal EJA: Pain begins in the dorsal horn—with a proposed classification of the primary senses. In: Crue BL (ed) Pain Research and Treatment. New York: Academic Press, 1975.
17. Crue BL, Kenton B, Carregal EJA: Review article—neurophysiology of pain—peripheral aspects. Presented at First World Congress on Pain, Sept. 7, 1975, Florence, Italy. (Sponsored by International Association for the Study of Pain.) In Crue BL (ed) Chronic Pain. New York: Spectrum, 1979. Also: Bull LA Neurol Soc 41:13–42, 1976.
18. Crue BL, Pinsky JJ, Agnew DC, Oliai R, Harth L: Observations on the taxonomy problem in pain. In: Chronic Pain—Further Observations. New York: Spectrum, 1979.
19. Agnew DC, Crue BL, Pinsky JJ: A taxonomy for diagnosis and information storage for patients with chronic pain. Bull LA Neurol Soc 44:84, 1979.
20. Crue BL, Kenton B, Carregal EJA, Pinsky JJ: The continuing crisis in pain research. In: Crue BL (ed) Chronic Pain. New York: Spectrum, 1979; and Smith WL, Merskey H, Gross SC (eds) Pain, Meaning and Management. New York: Spectrum, 1980.
21. Crue BL: Neurophysiology and taxonomy of pain. In: Brena S, Chapman S (eds) Management of Patients with Chronic Pain. New York: Spectrum, 1983.
22. Crue BL, Saltzberg B: Dynamic pain. Bull LA Neurol Soc 44:127, 1979.
23. Melzack R, Wall PD: Pain mechanisms: A new theory. Science 150:971, 1965.
24. Sternbach, RA: Pain: A Psychophysiological Analysis. New York: Academic Press, 1968.
25. Sternbach RA: Strategies and tactics in the treatment of patients with pain. In: Pain and Suffering —Selected Aspects. Springfield, Ill.: Charles C Thomas, 1970.
26. Casey K: Some current views on the neurophysiology of pain. In: Crue BL (ed) Pain and Suffering—Selected Aspects. Springfield, Ill.: Charles C Thomas, 1970, pp 168–175.
27. Crue BL: Comments on recent neurochemical central brain stem aspects of pain. In Chronic Pain. New York: Spectrum, 1979.
28. Crue BL: The centralist concept of chronic pain. Sem Neurol 3:331–339, 1983.
29. Brena SF, Crue BL, Stieg RL: Comments on the classifications of chronic pain: Its clinical significance. Bull Clin Neurosciences 49:67–81, 1984.
30. Crue BL: Foreword. In: Aronoff, GM (ed) Evaluation and Treatment of Chronic Pain. Baltimore-Munich: Urban & Schwarzenberg, 1985.
31. Crue BL: Neuritis, neuropathy, and neuralgia. Curr Concepts Pain 1:3–10, 1983.
32. Black R: Trigeminal pain. In: Pain and Suffering—Selected Aspects. Springfield, Ill: Charles C Thomas, 1970.

33. Crue BL: Multidisciplinary pain treatment programs—current status. J Clin Pain 1, 1985.
34. Shelden CH, Pudenz RH, Freshwater DB, Crue BL: Compression rather than decompression for trigeminal neuralgia. J Neurosurg 12:123–126, 1955.
35. Crue BL, Shelden CH, Pudenz RH, Freshwater DB: Observations on the pain and trigger mechanism in trigeminal neuralgia. Neurology 6:196–207, 1956.
36. Crue BL, Sutin J: Delayed action potentials in the trigeminal system of cats. J Neurosurg 16:477–502, 1959.
37. Carregal E, Crue BL, Todd EM: Further observations of trigeminal; antidromic potentials. J Neurosurg 20:277–288, 1963.
38. Crue BL, Carregal EA, Todd EM: Neuralgia: Consideration of central mechanisms. Bull LA Neurol Soc 29:107–132, 1964.
39. Todd EM, Crue BL, Vergadamo M: Conservative treatment of post herpetic neuralgia. Bull LA Neurol Soc 30:148–152, 1965.
40. Crue BL, Kilham OW, Carregal EJA, Todd EM, Peripheral trigeminal potentials. Bull LA Neurol Soc 32:17–29, 1967.
41. Crue BL, Todd EM, Carregal EJA, Kilham O: Percutaneous trigeminal tractotomy. Bull LA Neurol Soc 32:86–92, 1967.
42. Crue BL, Todd EM, Carregal EJA: Cranial neuralgia—neurophysiological considerations. Handbook of Neurology, vol 5, Amsterdam, 1968.
43. Crue BL, Todd EM, Carregal EJA: Observations on the present status of the compression procedure in trigeminal neuralgia. In Crue BL (ed) Pain and Suffering—Selected Aspects. Springfield, Ill: Charles C Thomas, 1970.
44. Crue BL, Felsoory A: Transcutaneous high cervical "electrical cordotomy." Minn Med J 57:204–209, 1974.
45. Kenton B, Crue BL, Carregal EJA: The role of cutaneous mechanoreceptors in thermal sensation and pain. Pain 2:119–140, 1976.
46. Crue BL, Carregal EJA: Postsynaptic repetitive neuron discharge in chronic neuralgic pain. Presented at the International Symoposium on Pain, May 29, 1973, Seattle, Washington. Adv Neurol 4:643–649, 1974.
47. Ramzy I, Wallerstein RS: Pain, fear, and anxiety. A study in their inter-relationships. Psychoanal Study Child 13:147, 1958.
48. Pinsky JJ: Psychodynamics and psychotherapy in the treatment of patients with chronic intractable pain. In Crue BL (ed) Pain: Research and Treatment. New York: Academic Press, 1975.
49. Pinsky JJ: Chronic intractable benign pain; a syndrome and its treatment with intensive short term group psychotherapy, J Human Stress 4:17, 1978.
50. Crue BL, Pinsky JJ: Chronic pain syndrome—four aspects of the problem: New Hope Pain Center and Pain Research Foundation. In: New Approaches to Treatment of Chronic Pain. Research # 36, Monograph Series, National Institute on Drug Abuse, May 1981.
51. Pinsky JJ: Psychodynamic understanding and treatment of the chronic intractable benign pain syndrome—treatment outcome. Sem Neurol 3:346, 1983.
52. Pinsky JJ, Crue BL: Intensive group psychotherapy. In: Wall PD, Melzack R (eds) Textbook of Pain. New York: Churchill Livingstone, 1984.
53. Long DM: Surgical therapy of chronic pain. Neurosurgery 6:317–28, 1980.
54. Fordyce WE: On interdisciplinary peers. Arch Phys Med Rehab 62:51, 1981.
55. Crue BL, Pinsky JJ, Agnew DC, Malyon AK, Felsoory A, Kenton B, Appuzzo M: What is a pain center? In: Crue BL (ed) Chronic Pain. New York: Spectrum, 1979. Also: Bull LA Neurol Soc 41:160–167, 1976
56. Bonica JJ: The Management of Pain. Philadelphia: Lea Febiger, 1953.
57. Bonica JJ, Black RG: The management of a pain clinic in relief of intractable pain. In: Swerdlow M (ed) Monograph in Anesthesiology #1. New York: Ercepta Medica, 1974, pp 116–129.
58. Bonica JJ: Organization and function of a pain clinic. In Bonica JJ (ed) Advances in Neurology (vol 4—International Symposium on Pain). New York: Raven Press, 1974, p 433.
59. Bonica JJ (ed): Preface. In: Vol 4, Advances in Neurology (International Symposium on Pain) New York: Raven Press, 1974.
60. Black RG: The chronic pain syndrome. Surg Clin N Am 55:999, 1975.
61. Black RG: The chronic pain syndrome. Clin Med 82:17, 1975.
62. Pinsky JJ, Griffin SE, Agnew DC, Kamdar MD, Crue BL, Pinsky LH: Aspects of long-term evaluation of pain unit treatment program for patients with chronic intractable benign pain syndrome: Treatment outcome. Bull LA Neuro Soc 44:53, 1979.

63. Pinsky JJ, Crue BL, Griffin S: Why a pain unit? In: Crue BL (ed). Chronic Pain. New York: Spectrum, 1979.
64. Crue BL: A role for a neurosurgeon on the pain unit. In: Crue BL (ed) Chronic Pain. New York: Spectrum, 1979.
65. Aronoff GM (ed): Evaluation and Treatment of Chronic Pain. Baltimore-Munich: Urban and Schwarzenberg, 1985.
66. Stieg RL, Williams RC: Chronic pain as a biosociocultural phenomenon: Implications for treatment. Sem Neurol 3:370, 1983.
67. Morse RH: Toward an eclectic stance in algology. Sem Neurol 3:355, 1983.
68. Todd EM, Crue BL, Carregal EJA: Posterior approach for high cervical cordotomy and trigeminal tractotomy. Confina Neurol 31:106–115, 1969.
69. Crue BL, Felsoory A: Analgesia from percutaneous periaqueductal gray electrical stimulation in the human. Presented at Second World Congress on Pain Research, Sept. 1, 1978. Montreal. In: Bonica J et al. (eds) Advances in Pain Research and Therapy, vol 3. New York: Raven Press, 1979.
70. Crue BL, Felsoory A, Agnew D, Kamdar MD, Randle W, Griffin S, Sherman R, Menard P, Pinsky JJ: The team concept in the management of pain in patients with cancer. Bull LA Neurol Soc 44:70, 1979.
71. Crue BL: Treatment of patients with pain due to cancer. In: Gross SC, Garbs (eds) Cancer Treatment and Research in Humanistic Perspective. New York: Springer, 1985.
72. Neal: The Politics of Pain. New York: McGraw-Hill, 1978.
73. Frank JD: Holistic medicine—a view from the fence. Johns Hopkins Med J 194:222–227, 1981.
74. Crue BL (ed): The present status of therapy for clinical pain states. In: Pain: Research and Treatment. New York: Academic Press, 1975.
75. Crue BL: Historical review—American Pain Society—in accreditation of pain clinics and pain centers (moderated by Aronoff G). Presented at American Pain Society meeting, Chicago, November 1983. (Published in vol 1 of J Amer Acad Algology.)
76. Altman S, Crue BL: What is a pain center—an organizational model. Presented at American Pain Society meeting, Chicago, November 11, 1983. (Published in vol 1 of J Amer Acad Algology.)
77. Crue BL: Overview of pain clinic survey. Presented on Panel on CARF Survey of Pain Centers (moderated by Nichols J). International Association for the Study of Pain meeting, Seattle, 1984. (Published Am J Algology.)
78. Time (cover story): Unlocking pain's secrets, June 11, 1984.
79. AMA: Guides to the Evaluation of Permanent Impairment 2nd ed. Chicago, 1984, p 73.
80. Lee J: Lemons from a shady dealer. Time May 23, 1983, p 60.

2. ORGANIZATION AND PERSONNEL FUNCTIONS IN THE PAIN CLINIC

GERALD M. ARONOFF AND PATRICIA W. MCALARY

THE PAIN TEAM AND GOALS

Chronic pain syndromes are among the most difficult medical problems to treat. The present use of this term refers to non-malignant pain in which the subjective pain complaints, resultant suffering, and pain behaviors are excessive and disproportionate to the actual pathophysiology. In addition, there is generally accompanying life disruption and maladaptive behavior patterns demonstrated by impairments in physical and psychosocial functioning. Since pain is influenced by physiological, psychosocial, ethnocultural, religious, and motivational factors, a multidisciplinary approach is often necessary to effectively intervene in this process.

The primary responsibility for pain management has traditionally been the physician's, utilizing a variety of medications and/or procedures in an inpatient or outpatient setting to interrupt the nociceptive process. Although in recent years we have witnessed major advances in the delivery of potent medications and sophisticated invasive procedures for acute and cancer pain, these techniques are often less useful in managing chronic nonmalignant pain syndromes. What has been shown to be effective is coordinated and integrated multidisciplinary and interdisciplinary team management. This involves physicians participating in treatment coordinated with dentists, nurses, psychologists, social workers, physical and occupational therapists, vocational counselors, and other health care personnel. Multidisciplinary pain centers (MPC), especially those with a strong behavioral orientation, most readily offer this type of treatment. [1]

There are many types of pain treatment facilities: modality-oriented (TENS, acupuncture, nerve blocks), often unidisciplinary; syndrome-oriented facilities (low back pain, headache, arthritis, temperomandibular joint dysfunction), occasionally unidisciplinary but generally multidisciplinary; and multidisciplinary pain centers that treat a heterogeneous population of pain patients. However, every organized group is not a "pain center." A comprehensive pain center is one that offers "multidisciplinary evaluation, treatment, and an integrated pain team approach, directed toward both modification of pain and drug seeking behavior and the interruption of the disability process."[2] It must therefore "address the medical, psychological, and social contributions to the pain problem, and be staffed by a group of health professionals with interest and experience in managing pain."[3] The treatment goals are agreed upon by the staff and shared with the patient. Table 2—1 lists the common goals of multidisciplinary pain centers.[1]

It is the MPC model that will be the focus of this chapter, and specific references will be made to our inpatient program, the Boston Pain Center (BPC) at Spaulding Rehabilitation Hospital (SRH).

Experience has demonstrated the importance of the multidisciplinary team approach in the treatment of chronic pain, especially when the etiology of the pain problem has eluded diagnosis and/or adequate management via conventional methods. In an attempt to widen the patient's choice of treatment modalities, pain centers have emerged as an effective way to manage chronic pain.[4] In an 18-month to 10-year follow-up study, Meilman et al. noted a statistically significant decrease in medication use, number of hospitalizations, surgeries, pain levels, litigation, and compensation in patients treated in this setting. Patients rated their disability, activity level, and ability to engage in social, recreational, and work activities.[5]

With the development of the MPC, emphasis has been directed away from the

Table 2–1. Goals of multidisciplinary pain centers

1. Improve pain control (eliminate pain if possible).
2. Through physical therapies,
   (a) Help the patient be more active more comfortably.
   (b) With individually structured exercise programs, reduce patient's fear of reinjury.
   (c) Teach proper body mechanics and postural awareness.
   (d) Evaluate limitations/restrictions.
3. Improve psychological functioning
   (a) Define and address psychosocial issues influencing chronic pain syndrome.
   (b) Treat depression and frequently associated insomnia.
   (c) Address primary and secondary gains.
   (d) Family assessment.
   (e) Strengthen support systems (e.g., personal and environmental resources).
4. Provide access to occupational/vocational rehabilitation (and any other significant health care personnel).
5. Communicate with the patient's private/clinical physician via discharge summary/phone/personal meetings any information that will assist in their continued management of the patient.

traditional medical model, which treats chronic pain as an extension of acute pain. The conventional approach of the medical model to pain intervention is that "most treatments are directed at the patient alone and seek to discover and alleviate the source of the presumed nociceptive stimulation."[2] Failure to recognize and treat the psychosocial aspects of chronic pain often contributes to the development of chronic pain syndromes. By definition, chronic nonmalignant pain syndromes differ from acute pain syndromes in the following ways[6]:

1. Acute pain is biologically useful and often reflective of an underlying disorder. In chronic pain syndromes, pain no longer serves an adaptive purpose and often becomes the disease.
2. Acute pain may require potent narcotics and is usually relieved when the nociceptive stimuli cease. Narcotics are generally inappropriate in treating chronic pain syndromes, and pain usually persists or recurs long after the original nociception ceases.

Bonica describes chronic pain as a "malefic force that imposes severe emotional, physical, economic, and social stresses on the patient, on the family, and on society."[7]

ADMINISTRATIVE STRUCTURE

Our inpatient pain center is autonomous in its functioning, yet governed by the administration (and medical bylaws) of the Spaulding Rehabilitation Hospital in which our 21-bed unit is housed. Each clinical specialty area at the BPC (e.g., physical therapy, nursing, social service) is directly responsible to the medical director of the pain center and also to its department head at SRH. The SRH is affiliated with both the Harvard and Tufts Medical schools, and the pain center is one resource for teaching. Although the pain center is not a required rotation, it is offered as an elective for medical students and medical/surgical house officers. Psychology and social work internships are also available, and nursing students from several university and hospital-based nursing schools utilize the pain center for observational clinical experience. It is our belief that no clinicians entering practice in which they will treat chronic pain patients should do so without the benefit of exposure to the multidisciplinary management of difficult chronic pain syndromes.

Most members of the treatment team are employees of the hospital, but they are selected by the medical director of the pain unit. The clinical/administrative assistant is directly employed by the director. Our location within the hospital provides for use of ancillary services (radiology, laboratory, pharmacy, dietary, occupational therapy, and a large, well-equipped physical therapy department), as well as many of our medical consultants and house officers for coverage of emergency situations. Although surgical and emergency room services are not available within our facility, they are readily accessible at an adjacent acute care hospital, the Massachusetts General Hospital.

THE MULTIDISCIPLINARY TEAM

Approaching chronic pain from the unique perspectives of its members, the multidisciplinary team functions as a coordinated and cohesive unit, addressing the multidimensional aspects of the patient's pain syndrome from a similar underlying philosophy. The cohesiveness of the team is especially important in dealing with the maladaptive pain behaviors that many chronic pain patients engage in, often sabotaging the treatment plan. The following services are the responsibility of the treatment team:

1. A thorough medical assessment of the pain complaints, including detailed review of previous evaluations and treatments to assure that pertinent workup or treatment options have been addressed. If further evaluation is needed, it is obtained. However, an MPC should not be viewed primarily as a diagnostic center since most patients have already been extensively evaluated. These diagnostic services should be utilized for testing deemed necessary if the pain evaluation is incomplete, results need further clarification, or for necessary management of ongoing medical problems.
2. Medical history and physical examination and monitoring of other medical problems.
3. Psychiatric and psychological evaluation, including testing, to determine pertinent underlying (prepain) and resultant (postpain) psychological problems, and coping styles that impact on the patient's chronic pain syndrome. Individual and group psychotherapy and education address the problem areas.
4. Social service evaluation and intervention, viewing pain as a systems problem, recognizing that although the patient is defined as the one having the problem, the family either covertly or overtly may complicate the patient's recovery. The family can also be the ally in implementing the treatment plan.
5. Physical therapy evaluation to assess structural limitation/restrictions (objective findings versus pain complaints), body mechanics and postural deviations, range of motion, strength, flexibility; teach pain control modalities, for example, TENS or ice massage); and maximize function.
6. Systematic relaxation training with biofeedback as indicated.
7. Primary nursing to coordinate the entire patient care plan (their work in the above areas, development of more productive coping strategies, overall health behaviors, and medication management).
8. Vocational assessment to determine whether a patient can return to a former job or requires retraining.

PERSONNEL

The director

The Commission on Accreditation of Rehabilitation Facilities (CARF) *Standards for Chronic Pain Management Programs* recommends assigned responsibility for program direction and medical direction (which need not be the same person). It also specifies that the program director need not be a physician. Although currently the vast majority of programs are physician directed, some are under the program direction of clinical psychologists, nurses, or social workers. However, there must be medical supervision of physician-prescribed services. CARF further recommends that the designated individual(s) have training and expertise in managing the chronic pain population.[8]

The medical director may have a subspecialty in a number of different areas—neurology, neurosurgery, orthopedics, physiatry, anesthesiology, psychiatry—depending on the type of pain treatment focus. However, the expertise, interest in, and philosophy of pain management are often more important than the area of specialization.

In our MPC the medical director, Gerald M. Aronoff, is also program director and administrator. Certified by the American Board of Psychiatry and Neurology and with fellowship training in psychosomatics, he has specialized in algology (pain management) full time for 11 years. Aronoff is actively involved in preadmission evaluation, determination of treatment philosophy and goals, evaluating patient progress, patient and staff education, and research.

The director evaluates all patients referred to the pain center (by physicians or other health care providers) to determine their appropriateness for the pain program and potential for return to productive functioning, despite physical illness or continuing pain. He reviews findings of past and current medical evaluations, formulates his current impressions, assesses need for any further evaluation, and evaluates patient commitment to participate in a pain program aimed at decreasing disability from pain. His impressions, plans for admission, or other recommendations for treatment are then communicated to the referral source. He defines and communicates the philosophy, structure, and rules and regulations of the program to the patient.

The director uses an objective, and when necessary, confrontative approach. He attempts to delineate the organic and functional components of the patient's pain syndromes, including conscious and unconscious secondary gain, maladaptive and self-defeating behavior patterns, and rigid defenses. This frequently generates anger in the patient, and often is a positive first step in destabilizing and eventually changing maladaptive behaviors built around somatization and suffering. The patient is then referred to individual therapists to work on the specific problem areas.[9] This approach is in contrast to the acute medical model, in which the patient is a passive recipient of care, usually without responsibility for active participation or change.

The director monitors individual patient progress in the program during medical rounds, held in a patient group forum with nursing and other team members. Issues addressed are tapering and discontinuation of analgesics and other medications, utilization of alternative pain control modalities (heat, ice massage, TENS, relaxation techniques, physical therapy), and progress in dealing with medical and psychosocial issues contributing to the pain syndrome. The director also participates in ongoing patient care and discharge planning by providing input at treatment conferences on a regular basis. He conducts patient education groups on topics related to chronic pain management—for example, medical impairment and disability, medications and chronic pain, pain behaviors, and secondary gain. Patients are seen in regular follow-up appointments postdischarge, and weekly pain psychotherapy groups are also conducted by the director. He is actively involved in clinical research and lecturing on issues related to multidisciplinary pain management.

The assistant to the director (clinical and administrative)

In our program, this position is held by a clinical specialist in nursing (Patricia McAlary, RN, MS); however, in different programs the discipline of the assistant may vary, based on the requirements of the role. At the BPC the clinical assistant functions in a liaison capacity between referral sources (physicians, agencies, vocational and rehabilitation specialists, attorneys, insurance carriers) and the pain center; between the treatment team, other consultants, and the director; and patients and the director. She evaluates patients referred to the pain center with the director and, via documentation of patient appropriateness and plan of care, is often involved in obtaining third-party authorization for admission to the program.

Once patients are admitted to the program, their progress in all therapies is monitored and documented. The assistant is involved in patient care conferences, medical rounds, and interacts closely with the treatment team to reinforce patient care goals. Responsibilities also include administrative representation of the director in his absence, carrying out the philosophy and policies noted earlier.

The clinical assistant also serves as a resource to the nursing staff, participates in education of colleagues and clinical research, and triages in-house pain consultations prior to evaluation by the director.

Team consultants

Medical physician

In this context, the term *medical physician* will refer to internists, family physicians, and general practitioners to distinguish them from psychiatrists or those in other medical specialties (surgery, anesthesiology, neurology, and so on).[10] The medical physician has a unique opportunity to enlist the patient's trust and confidence. When diagnostic impressions and treatment goals are being formulated during the initial phases of the pain program, medical physicians often have the most credibility to the patient because of their orientation toward pathophysiology and organic disease. The patient often views psychiatrists and psychologists with initial skepticism, feeling they attribute all symptomatology to psychological problems and overlook organic concerns. In fact, with most chronic pain patients, both mechanisms operate to varying degrees, and their specific impact on their chronic pain syndrome must be delineated.[10]

Since some chronic pain patients with multiple medical problems, somatic complaints, and treatment failures often have associated dysfunctional behavior, and a hostile and demanding attitude, the medical physicians must not only be astute diagnosticians, but also be patient and supportive in order to build an alliance, and at the same time be clear, firm, and straightforward in presenting formulations and findings to patients. They must also be able to assess the impact of characterological and psychosocial factors on patients' conditions. This requires close collaboration with the other health professionals on the team and is quite different from the sole responsibility for "curing" the patient, which they often have in acute medicine.[10]

Specifically, responsibilities begin with a complete medical history on each patient within 24 hours of admission. The medical physician carefully reviews the pain complaint (location, onset, duration, character, precipitating and relieving factors), all previous diagnostic and therapeutic encounters, and etiologic impressions. The importance of this sometimes tedious verbal and written review cannot be overemphasized. It serves a number of crucial functions:[10]

1. Development of a therapeutic relationship with a patient whose previous medical treatment has often been characterized by repeated, inconclusive testing, unsuccessful and even detrimental therapies, and rejection.
2. The formulation of an accurate assessment of the multiple factors contributing to the chronic pain syndrome and any further diagnostic tests or consultations that may be indicated.
3. Observation of the status of any ongoing medical problems and treatment.

Factors in the patient's history suggesting a major psychogenic component to the pain syndrome include psychosocial disruptions, multiple vague medical complaints, multiple medical providers, multiple treatment failures, and polypharmacy.[10]

The physical examination must carefully assess objective signs of impairment or dysfunction (versus exaggerated, voluntary, or nonanatomic distribution of symptoms). At various times throughout the patient's admission, follow-up examinations may be warranted to assess consistency of findings or to reassure the patient that a new or persistent pain complaint does not indicate a new or progressive process. Since the majority of these patients have already been extensively tested, the medical physician must be extremely judicious in ordering further laboratory screening, diagnostic testing, or consultations. This is a population prone to iatrogenic complications, and invasive studies are to be avoided unless clinically indicated. Many of our patients have pending litigation (workers' compensation or personal injury), for which conscious or unconscious primary or secondary gain is often an issue. With these patients it is especially important to determine that the diagnostic impressions are supported by appropriate data.

Patients frequently have a multitude of somatic complaints and long-standing, or new symptomatology other than their primary pain complaint. If at all possible, testing and treatment of these conditions should not interfere with their pain program. When patients are initially evaluated for the program, plans should be made to manage any conditions requiring extensive treatment prior to admission or postdischarge.

In our inpatient program the medical physician or covering physician is available 24 hours per day, 7 days per week as needed. Each patient's medical status is monitored throughout the program as indicated by his or her condition. Formal review is done weekly during walking rounds with the medical director, nursing staff, and other team members. In the medical director's absence, the medical physician or other medical consultants may provide coverage.

Psychiatrist

The psychiatric consultant in a multidisciplinary pain center must have a working knowledge of the psychodynamics of chronic pain syndromes, the psychological issues faced by these patients, and their characteristic personality structures. As patients present with various symptom complexes (e.g., somatoform disorders, psychological factors affecting physical condition, substance-abuse disorders, atypical depression), the psychiatrist must define, clarify, and document them for the staff and patient. This process begins with an initial pain psychiatric evaluation within 48 hours of admission, including formulation of Diagnostic Statistical Manual-III[11] diagnosis and delineation of pertinent psychosocial issues contributing to disability from pain, such as secondary gain, unmet dependency needs, somatized anxiety.

A combined psychotherapeutic approach is applied in our program, with the treatment director, as noted, taking a direct and confrontative approach regarding the need to eliminate maladaptive pain behaviors, and the psychiatrist conducting individual psychotherapy with ego-oriented and psychodynamic aspects.[9] The former "insists on compliance," the latter "establishes an alliance," empathizing with the patient's struggle with pain.[12] Individual sessions are weekly or more often if psychiatric issues warrant. The psychiatrist acknowledges the depressive reaction to chronic, intractable pain, also noting previous chronic depression in the patient and family history. Character analysis is utilized, with exploration of the patient's patterns of coping with all emotional events, rather than just specific situations, and orientation to feelings in general. Patients usually respond positively to this approach, which encourages them to gain insight about their behavior and attitudes and gradually learn an awareness of feelings and more direct and effective coping patterns than use of pain.[9]

One of the most difficult aspects of treating patients with chronic pain syndromes is their characteristic lack of psychological-mindedness on the one hand, and the overwhelming psychogenic overlay to their symptoms on the other. They tend to express their emotions and needs through their behavior, pain, and symptomatology, with stress expressed physiologically, through autonomic, vascular, or neuromuscular mechanisms (e.g., muscle contraction headaches, hypertension, palpitation). "Psychologically, they are rigidly defensive, and use denial, repression, and projection... and are unable to identify personal axioms, values, or beliefs related to major life issues."[12] These personality characteristics separate them from other psychologically healthy patients and warrant psychotherapy aimed at altering and enhancing coping strategies and building self-esteem and appropriate assertiveness and need fulfillment. In isolation, insight-oriented individual psychotherapy is generally not effective in their treatment.[13]

The psychiatrist also attempts to overcome basic mistrust of the health care system, resulting from multiple unsuccessful treatments, fragmentation, and rejection. The psychiatrist promotes cooperation with the program, focusing on the alliance of trust and motivation. This style, of course, is in contrast to the director's because the psychiatrist approaches the patient with nonjudgmental receptivity. Patients with complex, or refractory, psychiatric problems requiring specific pharmacological management often receive this from the psychiatrist.

Responsibilities of the psychiatrist also include crisis intervention including evaluation and treatment recommendations for patients who may be potentially or actually suicidal, aggressive, threatening, noncommunicative, noncompliant with the program, or severely regressed. This may involve patient referral to another setting, such as commitment to a psychiatric facility, if the psychiatric needs become the sole focus.

The psychiatrist also has teaching responsibility with the pain unit staff and meets formally with them on a weekly basis to address psychiatric issues involved in pain management (i.e., specific patients on the unit or more general pertinent topics). The psychiatrist is also a resource for the psychologists, psychology interns, and other staff.

Neurologist

At the BPC, the consulting neurologist has also had residency training in neurosurgery. His clinical experience and special interest in psychosomatic medicine assist the team in identifying patients who are likely to benefit from further neurodiagnostic study or treatment. Broad experience is necessary so that the consultant does not overreact to the patients' subjective complaints, which are frequently excessive and unsubstantiated by objective findings. We have found that many, if not most, of the patients who enter our pain center require neurologic consultation—for example to clarify the presence of true radiculopathy in cervical or lumbar pain syndromes, clarify headache variants, recommend medication management of neuropathic pain, and monitor treatment of patients' ongoing neurologic disorders (seizures, and so on).

In some facilities, neurologists may be responsible for performing electrodiagnostic studies. In our inpatient program this is the responsibility of the hospital's physiatry department. Our neurologic consultant also functions as an associate to the medical director, providing medical coverage in his absence and evaluating the appropriateness of new patients for the program.

Other consultants

As noted, chronic pain patients who enter the program have usually been extensively evaluated and reevaluated prior to their referral and admission. Repeat invasive tests to rule out organic pathology are likely to be conterproductive if (1) the previous accurate evaluation by the referring physician is negative, (2) appropriate consultations in the various subspecialties fail to reveal the nature of the pathology, and finally, (3) new tests are contraindicated in the opinions of consultants representing the MPC group.

Patient Care Coordinator

At the BPC, the patient care coordinator is a registered nurse, experienced in the care of chronic pain patients. She is an employee of the SRH, as are most other treatment team members, and is responsible to the director of nursing and hospital administration. However, she has a close working relationship with the director of the program to assure that the philosophy and goals of the MPC are implemented.

She manages all aspects of the functioning of the pain program and the interdisciplinary team. The nurses and other ancillary personnel are initially screened and interviewed by her, and all team members are directly responsible to her regarding patient care issues.

She coordinates scheduling of therapies and team meetings and assures that consistently high quality care is delivered. She is also responsive to patient concerns, consistently reiterating pain program policies, including the behavioral methodology.

Primary nurse

The primary nurse has at least two years of clinical experience and a commitment to holistic care and promotion of well-behavior. Recognizing the difference between acute and chronic pain management, she must refrain from the traditionally nurturant reactions to patients' pain complaints and pain behaviors—grimacing, groaning, limping, use of analgesics, supportive devices, drug-seeking behaviors. These passive responses to chronic pain are negatively reinforced (confronting or ignoring them), while active utilization of learned coping strategies and well-behaviors (participation in all therapies despite pain, independent use of pain control modalities such as ice massage, relaxation techniques) are positively reinforced (attentive listening, praise, physical contact such as hand shaking or hugging).[14]

The primary nurse must have an understanding of the physiological and psychosocial aspects of chronic pain syndromes, principles of behavior modification and operant conditioning, and medical-surgical nursing. Excellent clinical judgment is essential, since she is frequently faced with patients' multiple somatic complaints and must be astute in observing, evaluating, and differentiating pain behavior from medical symptomatology warranting further medical attention.

A thorough nursing pain assessment is essential and includes the following:

1. Pain history (pain pattern; onset; precipitating, aggravating, and relieving factors; treatments).

2. Medication history (pain and nonpain related, past and current substance abuse).
3. Medical history (including attention to stress-related disorders, health behaviors, frequency and appropriateness of use of the health care system).
4. Psychosocial history (marital, cultural, psychological depression and anxiety, family, developmental, "pain models," occupational such as job requirements, satisfaction, goals for return to work, compensation or disability issues).

Patients' initial appearances (affect, mental status, pain behavior) are noted, and changes monitored as patients progress through the program.[14]

In concluding her initial assessment, the nurse identifies problem areas, such as maladaptive behavior patterns, stressors, and current limitations related to pain. Together with the patient, measurable short and long-term goals are set and documented in the patient's record. A problem-oriented care plan is formulated, emphasizing the use of active alternative pain control methods and coping strategies rather than treatments to be to the patient. A supportive, trusting relationship is established. It is important that patients not have to prove the reality of their pain to the nurse. The patient's progress is monitored and reinforced by the primary nurse. Manipulative behavior can often be aimed at "splitting" the staff, that is, using pain to avoid activities. These issues are redirected through the primary nurse, who emphasizes the patient's responsibility for active participation and goal achievement in all areas of the program.[14]

The primary nurse is responsible for medication administration and education. Polydrug dependency and drug-seeking behavior are significant problems for many patients, who often enter the program taking narcotics, barbiturates, sedative hypnotics, anxiolytics, muscle relaxants, anti-inflammatory medications, and multiple over-the-counter or prescribed medications for other medical conditions. The pain program uses a number of methods to reduce patients' medication dependency. Although prescribed by the medical director, nursing is responsible for implementation of the following:

1. Eliminating on-demand medications for pain, with set medication times.
2. Gradually tapering and discontinuing medications as the patient utilizes alternative pain control modalities, copes better with stress, anxiety, depression, pain, and addresses issues contributing to them.
3. Patients obtaining medications at the nursing station.

Education in the proper use of medications is essential and requires frequent reinforcement. This is especially true regarding the use of tricyclic antidepressants in the management of the triad of chronic pain, depression, and insomnia, since these patients often vehemently deny their depression, relate insomnia only to pain, and have difficulty accepting elimination of other drugs and the use of an antidepressant. The nurse also plays a key role in other areas of patient education and health care management (weight loss, exercise and activity, nonsmoking), management of concurrent medical problems, and reinforcement of the work being done in other areas of the program.

Pain rehabilitation associate

At the BPC, pain rehabilitation associates (PRAs) are treatment team members who assist the nursing staff in their patient care, the physical therapists with pain control techniques (e.g., ice massage, oil massage), and the psychologists with relaxation and biofeedback instruction. They also act as facilitators in some psychotherapy groups.

As treatment team members, their effective use of communication skills, behavior modification techniques, and crisis intervention strategies is essential in their interactions with patients. They must be high school graduates with a minimum of two years education in human services. A bachelor's degree in social sciences and prior experience in stress management or psychology is preferred. Nursing assistant experience or Red Cross certification in first aid is also required.

Physical therapist

Our physical therapists work exclusively with pain patients (they are not assigned to other areas of the hospital). They must be graduates of an accredited school of physical therapy, and at least one year of clinical experience is preferred. Astute assessment skills are necessary to clearly distinguish pain behavior from actual dysfunction. Therapists must be supportive and understanding of patients' fears, yet able to "push" patients when necessary to help them increase their functional level.[15]

The goals of the physical therapy program are as follows:

1. Evaluation of the patient's musculoskeletal status (structure, function, alterations) and determination of goals, limitations, and restrictions.
2. Education of the patients regarding their functional goals, exercise program, postural corrections, and training in body mechanics.
3. Utilization of pain control modalities (e.g., TENS, ice massage, heat, whirlpool, untrasound, HVDC (high-voltage direct current).

Within 72 hours of the patient's admission a thorough physical therapy evaluation is completed detailing structure, function, pain complaint(s), use of assistive devices, and observation of affect and pain behavior. Pertinent musculoskeletal and neurologic findings are noted and correlated with anatomic dysfunction, previous treatments, and surgeries. The evaluation report includes pertinent physical findings, problem areas, specific goals, and treatment plan. Emphasis is placed on techniques the patient can utilize independently. An individualized and supervised exercise program for increasing strength, flexibility, range of motion, and endurance is a key part of the rehabilitative program. A group exercise class is held several times weekly, as well as weekly pool exercise session and a group "walk" to increase endurance and cardiovascular fitness.

The major goal of the exercise program is to help patients become more active, more comfortable with reduced risk of reinjury, and to teach them that hurt does not necessarily mean harm. Any specific structural limitations or restrictions (or the lack thereof) affecting the patient's return to work are addressed. Sometimes this may need to be clarified by orthopedic and/or neurologic consultation to rule out structural pathology since some patients are reluctant to relinquish pain as a disability even in the absence of supporting objective data. This is especially true with industrial accident patients when litigation is pending. Specific limitations and work recommendations or precautions are made known to the patient and are part of the discharge summary. Patients are discharged on a home exercise program in order to maintain their progress. Few require ongoing formal physical therapy unless indicated for another underlying or chronic condition (e.g., multiple sclerosis, paraplegia).

Psychologist

There are two clinical psychology positions, both at the Ph.D. level, with co-directorship of the biopsychology component. The term *biopsychology* was chosen because work with these patients necessarily involves helping them make the integral connection between their psychosocial problems and their somatic complaints (anxiety, depression, anger, unmet dependency needs, stress, tension, and pain).

The psychologists share the responsibility for leading psychotherapy group sessions in which issues pertinent to pain, stress management, and coping style are discussed. A weekly relaxation training group is led by the psychologists, and biofeedback services are coordinated by them. They conduct weekly educational groups on chronic pain as well as Saturday workshops on the psychophysiology of pain. Patients are seen on an individual basis as needed; this is coordinated with the psychiatrist and social worker to avoid duplication of services and confusion for the patient. Psychologists are also available for crisis intervention as needed. Thorough documentation in each patient's medical record reports progress in psychotherapy groups, relaxation sessions, and individual appointments. Psychologists also function in a supervisory capacity for PRAs doing relaxation and biofeedback training. There is a formal training program for psychology interns, who are supervised by the psychologists. Less formal supervision and resource assistance is provided to nursing and other staff members regarding psychological aspects of patient management.

As team members, the psychologists play an integral role in weekly patient care conferences, discharge planning meetings, and psychiatric conferences led by the consulting psychiatrist. They are also responsible for psychological testing on each patient. Currently, our tools include the Profile of Mood States (POMS), the McGill Pain Questionnaire (MPQ), and the Chronic Pain Battery (CPB). Based on individual patient indications, a full battery of neuropsychological testing may be done. We are in the process of reevaluating our current testing and are further developing a psychological pain profile.

Social worker

The social worker should have a Masters in Social Work (MSW) or licensed Social Work (LICSW) degree from an accredited school of social work, at least one year of postgraduate work experience, preferably in a clinical setting, and an interest in working with chronic pain patients and doing family therapy.

A thorough psychosocial, personal, family, and work history is essential, with assessment of stressors that may contribute to the patient's pain and disability. Developmental history is often significant for pain-prone disorders (e.g., traumatic childhood with unmet dependency needs, history of abuse or neglect, family history of alcoholism, psychiatric disturbances, pain and disability[16], in which the patient has functioned reasonably well until the onset of pain, at which time the patient's unconscious response is "now take care of me." Sources of interpersonal and family conflicts are identified and explored in regular individual and family meetings. The frequency of these meetings is dictated by the extent of the problems and the motivation of patient and family to address issues. Many out-of-state referrals necessitate telephone conferences with spouses and family members unable to attend a meeting. Issues addressed are coping styles, family dynamics, conscious and unconscious secondary gain from pain, and alteration of family roles and relationships related to the pain. Often patients and families have great difficulty facing these issues and create many obstacles to avoid doing so. Some common obstacles are denial of conflicts or need for change, unwillingness to involve spouse or significant family members, pretense of planned changes in relationships that do not occur, and refusal of postdischarge therapy.[17]

At least one-third of our patients are on workers' compensation or have pain-related litigation pending. There are multiple areas of potential secondary gain (e.g., monetary compensation through litigation, a "way out" of a disliked job, an acceptable disability allowing the patient to be taken care of). Objective assessments of structural or functional limitations and restrictions by other team members and consultants are reviewed, and appropriate vocational options are explored, with the goal of return to gainful employment, if not at the previous job, then at an alternative one. For some patients—in particular those who are older, retired, involved in child-rearing, or who choose other pursuits—involvement in the work force is not a realistic option. The social worker explores other options with them, and specific discharge plans are formulated. This often includes increased socialization for the elderly and those previously isolated due to pain (e.g., volunteer work, senior citizens' clubs, and other activity groups).

Vocational counseling is an important component in the MPC approach. The social worker facilitates these referrals when indicated. Many patients who enter our program are already working with rehabilitation or vocational counselors, who are kept apprised of their progress in the program and discharge planning.

For many patients, discharge planning includes referral for follow-up psychotherapy or counseling (individual, group, marital, or vocational). Most patients are discharged to their homes independent of services; however, any who require transfer to another facility or provision of home services have arrangements facilitated by the social worker. The social worker also conducts a weekly evening group meeting for educating patients and their families. Former patients often participate in these meetings as facilitators.

PAIN CENTER FUNCTIONS

The referral process

Patients are evaluated for admission to the pain center on a referral basis. Each year, more physicians and other health care providers are recognizing the MPC as a community resource and referring patients with disabling pain earlier in their pain careers rather than as a last resort. Patients are referred by orthopedists, rheumatologists, neurologists, neurosurgeons, anesthesiologists, internists, psychiatrists, psychologists, vocational and rehabilitation counselors, and many other medical subspecialists. Of the small percentage of patients who are self-referred, we ask that they obtain medical records from a treating physician for our review.

Many patients have musculoskeletal pain, with low back and cervical pain syndromes the most common, although intractable headaches and neuropathic, causalgic, rheumatic, cardiac, and gastroenterologic pain are also frequently encountered.[1] About one-third of our patients have had industrial accidents, another third nonwork-related personal injuries, and the remaining third have pain secondary to a disease process or medical condition (osteoporosis with compression fractures, systemic lupus erythematosis, chronic recurrent pancreatitis, diabetic neuropathy, phantom limb pain, to name a few). Of this latter group, pain is often disproportionate to the degree of organic pathology or uncharacteristic of that disease process (e.g., persistent postthoracotomy chest wall pain, in which intercostal neuritis, neuroma, and other etiologies have been excluded; non-ischemic chest pain in an anxious patient with known cardiac disease, inappropriately using nitroglycerine). Many patients have multiple and diffuse pains of obscure etiology and have undergone numerous invasive procedures, sometimes performed more at the patient's insistance than because of the physician's belief that they are warranted or likely to relieve pain.

Characteristics common in these patients include inordinate preoccupation with somatic complaints, passive-dependent personality traits, denial of past and current psychosocial conflicts, inability to deal effectively with emotions such as anger and hostility, and lack of insight into the inter-relationship between these and their pain problems.[1] A sub-group have a developmental history significant for pain-prone disorder.[16] Their past and current relationships are often characterized by self-defeating behaviors, such as abuse by spouses with resultant low self-esteem, and focus on pain as a method of having their needs met.

Economic factors often complicate their rehabilitative process, especially for patients currently receiving workers' compensation or other disability payments. They may feel they stand to gain more by remaining "disabled" by pain than by recovery and return to gainful employment, especially those patients who have little education, menial jobs, and difficult psychosocial histories, who sometimes

Table 2–2. Some characteristics of a sample of consecutive chronic pain patients admitted to Boston Pain Center (N = 76)

Characteristic	Data
Age	46.98 years
Education	12.94 years
Chronicity	4.67 years
Surgeries for pain	1.29
Number of medical appointments for pain during year before admission	17.87 appointments
Number taking narcotic medications	42 (55%)
Number of patients with a history of psychiatric disorders in the family	30 (40%)

feel "the system owes me something." Our experience indicates that those who remain disabled by pain and are unproductive tend to suffer more from continuing depression and decreased self-esteem, in contrast to those who return to some type of productive work or activity, despite any remaining pain. Our philosophy is that a person is rarely totally and permanently disabled, although returning to a previous, physically demanding job may not be feasible.

Demographic data on a recent group of 76 consecutive patients admitted to the BPC is included in table 2–2. Approximately 36 percent of our inpatients are referred from out of state, and we have treated a significant number of patients from outside the United States.[1]

When a patient is referred, it is not enough for the physician to want the patient to change. The patient himself must be motivated. Some patients wish to continue being cared for. They may do well within the milieu of the pain center but fail to utilize what they have learned. In addition to individual motivation, we have found that key predictors of patient success are effective support systems (family, friends, school, job, hobbies, community activities) and well-defined goals, or reasons to get better. Our experience has demonstrated that these factors have much more to do with success than diagnosis on admission, amount or type of medication, or previous surgeries or procedures.

The way the patient views referral to a pain center often depends on the referring physician's presentation of the suggestion. Several frequent misconceptions should be dispelled:

1. That pain centers are for people whose pain is all psychological. This is not the case, although patients with chronic pain syndromes do often have a complex interaction between physiological and psychological factors.
2. That chronic pain is necessarily disabling. Many patients leave complaining less of pain, some without pain, and for most, there is significantly diminished suffering and pain behavior; the majority of patients at discharge do not find their pain to be disabling.
3. That patients with chronic pain should be maintained on analgesics. The vast majority can be taught effective alternative pain-control techniques and, by

discharge from an MPC, suffer less not taking analgesics than they did on admission taking analgesics.

It should be carefully explained to the patients that a pain center referral is not "a last resort" but a specialized, comprehensive approach to exploring and treating the multiple aspects of their pain problem, which has now become the disease and is not resolving.[1]

Preadmission screening

Referred patients are asked to make the evaluation appointment themselves rather than having the referring physician's office do so, as the initial step in assessing their motivation and decreasing their dependent behavior patterns. They are initially evaluated by the clinical assistant, who reviews pertinent medical records, pain history and complaints, diagnostic evaluations, treatments and their effectiveness, medications, medical, family, psychosocial history, the degree of life disruption related to pain, and motivation for recovery. Patients must complete an extensive pain questionnaire prior to this evaluation, which addresses these areas. The patient, any family members present, and the clinical assistant then review all pertinent findings and pain history with the director, who continues the evaluation to determine appropriateness for the pain program or recommends other treatment options.

Inpatient MPC admission is indicated for those patients with global life disruption, severe depression often of suicidal proportions, major medication dependency, and other medical problems requiring inpatient monitoring. In addition, patients whose home situations, significantly contribute to their pain syndromes, those who are not ambulatory, or those who have already attempted outpatient pain treatment unsuccessfully are often best treated in an inpatient setting. A multidisciplinary, comprehensive day-treatment outpatient program is appropriate for many patients who have not had thorough outpatient modalities, do not have major medication dependency, and need to remain at home due to child care and other responsibilities. If they live too far from the center, arrangements can often be made for temporary lodging at a local hotel.

Advantages of outpatient treatment are reduced cost to patients or third-party payers, incorporation of routine daily activity such as driving to and from the program, and simulation of a more normalized daily routine. However, disadvantages include less control over patient attendance at the program. Patients bedridden due to pain can be confronted by the inpatient treatment team regarding lack of participation, while outpatients will often call in sick. Medication management is often more difficult in the outpatient setting, as is behavior modification, since at the end of the day patients often return to an environment that reinforces pain behavior. Although milieu therapy occurs at good day-treatment programs, for many patients it is not as intense as that provided in the inpatient setting.

For some chronic pain patients with only minimal life disruption (e.g., able to work, attend school), and who have had little outpatient pain treatment but require multidisciplinary management, a less intense but structured outpatient evening program is often an option, for example, several evenings per week. This schedule allows them to continue with their normal daily responsibilities yet affords them the benefit of the multidisciplinary approach to chronic pain treatment. This is often more effective than nonintegrated individual therapies, which lack a holistic approach by a cohesive pain team.

A smaller group of patients may present to the pain center with a pain problem that has not been thoroughly evaluated diagnostically or adequately treated. Further referral is then indicated. It is important that the patient not be asked to learn to live with pain that can be eliminated by an appropriate treatment. Examples of conditions amenable to treatment include the early states of postherpetic neuralgia before sympathetic nerve block and significant spinal instability secondary to a severe spondylolisthesis requiring further orthopedic or neurosurgical evaluation. However, the importance of a thorough review of the patient's pain, medical and psychosocial history, and behavior patterns during the evaluation cannot be overemphasized. Such a review clearly defines pertinent factors influencing pain-related disability and the most appropriate approach to overall patient management and requires a clinician experienced in chronic pain management.

Following the initial evaluation, the director makes telephone contact with the referral source to communicate the formulation and treatment plan. An extensive evaluation note follows that summarizes the information reviewed, documents the patient's life disruption, lists pertinent contributory factors from the patient's psychosocial and developmental history, and delineates the recommended treatment plan.

Once the patient is determined to be appropriate for either the inpatient or outpatient program, contact is made with health insurance carriers to obtain authorization for payment. Most provide coverage for inpatient and outpatient pain treatment. However, each plan is different, and coverage must be determined on an individual basis. Managed care and health maintenance organizations (HMOs) usually require preauthorization prior to admission, necessitating their review of the patient's history, prior pain therapies, and documentation of the need for comprehensive MPC management, especially when inpatient admission is planned. Patients receiving workers' compensation require prior approval from the insurance carrier, which often necessitates contact with the patient's attorney when litigation is pending. Our inpatient facility (SRH) requires written reimbursement authorization prior to admission. With current changes in the health care delivery system—diagnostic related groups (DRGs), increased requirements for cost effectiveness, documentation of necessity for provision of care—we have been faced with more stringent requirements to specify and document results of our program goals and treatment.

Admission diagnoses

Since 1972, we have seen more than seven thousand pain referrals, about half of whom have been admitted to the pain center. Cancer pain syndromes are treated elsewhere in the hospital.

DSM III diagnoses most frequently encoutered are atypical depression (reactive to pain and life disruption, sometimes with superimposed chronic features), anxiety disorders (usually characterized as somatized anxiety), psychological factors affecting physical condition, dysthymic disorder, and substance abuse disorder. Less frequently, psychogenic pain disorder, somatization disorder, and personality disorder are seen. It is extremely important to substantiate and document the diagnosis with appropriate clinical evidence so that patients are not diagnosed inaccurately or merely by exclusion. As indicated, some patients may enter the program extremely depressed with associated suicidal ideation. They are evaluated by the consulting psychiatrist to determine whether or not they are an acute risk (if so, they generally must be transferred to a psychiatric facility).

Monitoring patient progress

An individualized patient care plan with specific short and long-term goals is established on admission by each team member in collaboration with the patient. Progress toward these goals is documented in the medical record and discussed by the team in weekly patient care conferences.

In addition to the weekly treatment team conference and ongoing patient and therapist review of goals and objectives, a discharge planning meeting is held at approximately the midpoint of the four-to five-week program to review the patient's progress and reassess goals for the remaining portion of the program and for discharge. Discharge plans often include referrals for outpatient individual, group, marital, and vocational counseling in order to continue with gains made in the program in these areas. The discharge planning meeting is led by the medical director, and includes the patient, the entire treatment team, and significant family members when possible. With the patient's permission, the rehabilitation nurse or counselor and/or insurance representative may also attend. This may be especially important to patients on workers' compensation. Each therapist gives the patient a verbal progress report, discussing remaining goals and recommendations. The director summarizes overall progress since initial evaluation and any revisions in the treatment plan. All information, including a written summary, is documented in the patient's medical record.

The director leads several weekly evening pain psychotherapy groups for former patients. There is also a non-profit support organization known as Pain Copers for individuals suffering from chronic pain, which meets one evening a month at the hospital. This organization, founded in 1978 by GMA, espouses goals consistent with the philosophy of the pain center, namely provision of a support network of chronic pain sufferers and a forum for sharing adaptive ways of coping with pain.

In one of the weekly patient therapy groups led by the director, he reviews with the patient community the general progress and discharge meeting impressions of the team regarding the patients reviewed that week. The patient community is encouraged to provide constructive criticism directly to them at this time. For the patients, both their gains, as well as areas they must continue to address, are often reinforced.

At discharge, necessary referrals are formalized, including psychotherapy, vocational counseling, medical, sometimes a visiting nurse or home health aid and physical therapy. Patients are usually discharged on an independent home exercise program that incorporates the pain control modalities they have learned. They rarely require formal follow-up physical therapy, except in the isolated conditions noted. A discharge summary is sent to the referral source and any other physicians or health care providers specified by the patient who will be involved in follow-up care. The summary contains the reason for referral, discharge diagnoses —which often differ from diagnostic impressions on referral and admission— services provided, and patient progress, referrals, and interventions to be used by the patient and family to maintain gains and/or improve discharge functioning and increase independence. Follow-up appointments with the director are scheduled for one month postdischarge, then every three months the first year, every six months the second year, then yearly, unless the pain problem resolves. At follow-up, the patient completes a brief form of the preadmission questionnaire, which is used to obtain follow-up comparison data regarding life disruption related to pain and functional levels. Of the 76 former patients sampled in table 2–2, 50 percent in-state and 40 percent out-of-state returned for follow-up.

Program evaluation

To evaluate the progress of the BPC in meeting its stated goals and to determine which patients can be best served by the pain program, we are in the process of an ongoing quality assurance evaluation as part of our clinical research. The entire interdisciplinary team is participating, and rating scales for patient improvement in specific areas of functioning in response to interdisciplinary treatment are being assessed.

Follow-up studies of multidisciplinary pain centers

During the past 14 years numerous follow-up studies have attempted to determine the success of pain center programs. Typical problems in this research to date include "lack of comparison and control groups, use of self-report measures rather than more objective methods of assessing outcome, use of outcome measures with questionable validity and reliability, failure to use standardized instruments, lack of corroboration of self-reports, inadequate sample sizes, and dependence on mailed questionnaires."[18]

In order to proceed with effective and reliable research in this area, these problems must be addressed. Experts in the field must collaborate to determine the specific factors that indicate improvement and to develop standardized outcome measurements. In the interim, tests such as the McGill Pain Questionnaire, Profile of Mood States, Pilowski Illness Behavior Questionnaire, and the Sickness Impact Profile may be helpful, as well as other tests of vocational and psychosocial functioning.[18]

In regard to appropriate comparison groups, several suggestions include: patients who complete the program versus those who leave against medical advice and those who are treated in the program versus those who are appropriate for treatment but do not enter the program due to technical reasons (e.g., lack of insurance coverage). Another area of difficulty includes studies that attempt to compare results of pain programs varying greatly in their treatment approach, for examples, multidisciplinary pain centers versus unidisciplinary, such as anesthesiology pain services utilizing primarily nerve blocks. More valid comparisons might be made by groupings such as medically versus behaviorally oriented and inpatient versus outpatient.[18]

In an unpublished pilot study by Aronoff et al. of the BPC, in which 206 questionnaires were mailed to patients within a follow-up period between three months and one year, 75 questionnaires were returned. Results indicated that

57.5% of the respondents stated that their pain bothered them "not at all" to "moderately." Only 41.3% had used any pain medications, and of those, only 5% used narcotics. Only 25% were limited "quite a bit" or "extremely" by their pain. 75% reported "not at all" or "a little" to feelings of depression, anger, feeling tense. 86.6% had been out of their homes and 87.8% had been with other people "moderately" to "extremely." 45.3% were working (however, these figures are conservative since some respondents were housewives, retired, or for similar reasons not expected to be part of the work force), Social functioning improved in 59% of patients in relation to their families, 69% with friends, and 65% in their ability to fulfill familial duties. 74% of the sample reported continuation of their physical exercise program. 68.1% practiced relaxation exercises daily. 60% of those responding spent no time lying down due to pain and 25%, 2 hours lying down due to pain. 46.5% reported no pain-related medical encounters related to pain, and 12.3% had 3 or more medical visits.[18]

SPATIAL CONSIDERATIONS

Both the BPC at SRH and the out patient day treatment program, at the North Shore Pain Center (NSPC) in Peabody, Massachusetts, have about 2,500 square feet of space. The latter is a freestanding pain center utilizing one wing (floor) of the hospital. Two teams of seven patients can be treated at any given time at the NSPC.

Several spatial considerations are important for inpatient or outpatient treatment. An autonomous space should be utilized to promote milieu therapy. In the inpatient setting our 21 beds are on one wing of a hospital floor. When it is possible to have a distinct geographical area for the pain program, it is preferable.

It is helpful to have an open, centralized "nursing station" space where the program secretary and other support staff can be available. The station can incorporate areas for medical records, desk space for charting, message center, and so on. Accessible yet individual staff offices are essential for individual meetings with the patients and families, so that confidentiality can be maintained, as well as a quiet and undisturbed place for telephone access and dictation.

Separate exercise facilities are preferable. In both the inpatient and outpatient centers there is a small physical therapy examination room. An all-purpose group meeting room is used for group exercise classes. Since both centers are housed in hospitals, use of the larger physical therapy department with its more sophisticated equipment is possible.

At least one large group meeting room is necessary. It should have adequate sound proofing so that patients may freely discuss confidential issues without fear of being overheard. In addition, patients should have a room or area for socialization, with a comfortable and relaxed decor, possibly TV or radio, with allowances made for smoking and nonsmoking areas, although smoking is strongly discouraged. In our inpatient center, a large dining room is available (and also used as a group meeting room), with a separate room for socialization. The latter is the only place smoking is allowed on the pain unit. TV is available both in the dining room and the recreational room but is intentionally not provided in the patients' rooms (which are semi-private) to avoid social isolation and promote interaction and support among the community.

CONCLUSION

It is hoped that pain centers will no longer be viewed as a treatment of last resort. As this chapter suggests, no one discipline in isolation can possibly duplicate services provided by a multidisciplinary pain team. Medical direction for a pain team may be provided by a variety of disciplines; most important is the clinical experience of physicians, their dedication to treating chronic pain syndromes, and their ability to be part of a team. The physician's leadership is vital, but so are treatments provided by the other clinicians. On a good pain treatment team all are well trained and dedicated, working together synergistically for the patient's benefit.

REFERENCES

1. Aronoff GM , Wagner JM: Pain Centers: A Community Resource. Mediguide to Pain. Lawrence DellaCorte Publications Inc., 7:1 1–2, 1986.
2. Aronoff GM: The role of the pain center in the treatment of intractable suffering and disability resulting from chronic pain. Sem Neurol 3:4, December 1983.
3. Aronoff GM, Wagner JM: The pain center: development, structure, and dynamics. In: Handbook of Chronic Pain Management. Burrows, Elton, Stanley (eds) New York: Elsevier Science (Biomedical Division), 1987.pp 407–424
4. Aronoff GM: A holistic approach to pain rehabilitation: the Boston Pain Unit. In: Ng LKY (ed) New Approaches to Treatment of Chronic Pain: A Review of Multidisciplinary Pain Clinics and Pain Centers. Washington D.C.: National Institute of Drug Abuse, Research Monograph Series 36, May 1981, pp 33–40.
5. Meilman W, Skultety FM, Guck TP, Sullivan K: Benign chronic pain: 18 month to ten year follow-up of a multidisciplinary pain unit treatment program. Clin J Pain 1:3, 131–137, 1985.
6. Aronoff GM: Psychological aspects of non-malignant chronic pain: a multidisciplinary approach. Resident and Staff Physician, 1984, pp 3–14.

7. Bonica JJ: U.S. Department of Health, Education and Welfare: Report of the Panel on Pain to the National Advisory Neurological and Communicative Disorders and Stroke Council, May 3, 1980.
8. Standards Manual for Organizations Serving People with Disabilities. Commission on Accreditation of Rehabilitation Facilities. Tuscon, Arizona, 1986, pp 46–47.
9. Aronoff GM, Rutrick D: Psychodynamics and psychotherapy of the chronic pain syndrome. In: Aronoff GM (ed) Evaluation and Treatment of Chronic Pain. Baltimore: Urban & Schwarzenberg, 1985, pp 463–469.
10. Savitz D: Medical evaluation of the chronic pain patient. In: Aronoff GM (ed) Evaluation and Treatment of Chronic Pain. Baltimore: Urban & Schwarzenberg, 1985, pp 39–60.
11. Diagnostic Criteria from DSM III. The American Psychiatric Association. Washington, D.C., 1980.
12. Rutrick D, Aronoff GM: Combined psychotherapy for chronic pain syndrome patients at a multidisciplinary pain center. In: Aronoff GM (ed) Evaluation and Treatment of Chronic Pain. Baltimore: Urban & Schwarzenberg, 1985, pp 485–493.
13. Merskey H: Pain and personality. In: Sternback R (ed) The Psychology of Pain. New York: Raven Press, 1978, pp 111–127.
14. Sample S, Page MB, Hayes M: Chronic pain management: the nurse's role. In: Aronoff GM (ed) Evaluation and Treatment of Chronic Pain. Baltimore: Urban & Schwarzenberg, 1985, pp 563–564.
15. Yeh C, Gonyea MB, Lemke J, Volpe M: Physical therapy. In: Aronoff GM (ed) Evaluation and Treatment of Chronic Pain. Baltimore: Urban & Schwarzenberg, 1985, pp 251–261.
16. Blumer D: Psychiatric and psychological aspects of chronic pain. Clin Neurosur 25:276–283, 1978.
17. Goldberg P: The social worker, family systmes, and the chronic pain family. In Aronoff GM (ed) Evaluation and Treatment of Chronic Pain. Baltimore: Urban & Schwarzenberg, 1985, pp 571–587.
18. Aronoff GM. Evans WO, Enders PL: A review of follow-up studies of multidisciplinary pain units. In: Aronoff GM (ed) Evaluation and Treatment of Chronic Pain. Baltimore: Urban & Schwarzenberg, 1985, pp 511–521.

3. MULTIDISCIPLINARY APPROACHES TO THE MANAGEMENT OF CHRONIC PAIN

JOHN C. ROWLINGSON AND TIMOTHY C. TOOMEY

Pain management has become increasingly more popular since Melzack and Wall's Gate Control Theory made it plausible that pain could exist without injury and be absent in the presence of injury.[1] A great deal of research was triggered by their theory, and worldwide interest in pain mechanisms, multidisciplinary evaluation protocols, and management techniques escalated. As the search for more reliable evaluation approaches and treatment modalities paid off, and as our understanding of the complexity of pain grew, more medical and scientific specialists have necessarily become involved in pain management. Patients have also become more knowledgeable about what is available in pain control. In this day and age of consumer advocacy, the views of the public cannot be ignored. It is vital, then, that pain be accurately diagnosed and effectively treated, not only because of its pathophysiologic impact and its adverse effects on morbidity and mortality, but also because of its contribution to incalculable agony and suffering.

By demand and of necessity, an increasing number of health care specialists must become more knowledgeable not only about the fundamentals of patient evaluation for various kinds of pain problems, but also about the scientific mechanisms that subserve the vast experience called "pain" and the therapeutic modalities that logically may be used. No longer can specialists narrowly view patients considering only the treatment their specialty training provides. If specialists cannot or will not broaden their attitude toward patient evaluation and treatment, other consultants must participate in patients' workup and treatment programs. Only with this integrated, contemporary approach will successful treatment be most likely. Some specialists have found it exceedingly beneficial and efficient to organize themselves into pain centers and pain clinics whereby the multidisciplinary approach to the management of chronic pain is maximally manifest.

While the demands for proper care of patients are high, there are a number of valid reasons why one might choose not to become involved with patients who have problems with chronic pain (see table 3–1). A busy practice situation may preclude keeping up to date with advances in pain management, let alone allowing time to evaluate or treat patients as the new concepts dictate. The very nature of a chronic condition implies difficulty in finding effective treatment that patients will follow with enough consistency to test its effectiveness. Thus, physicians and others involved in the care of patients with chronic pain can easily become discouraged and frustrated with the lack of success, emotions that may be shared by patients. Even when treatment of pain is successful, the complaints may persist or be amplified by pressing psychosocial issues or the complexities of our present legal and/or compensation systems.

The multidisciplinary approach to pain management distributes the time requirement and responsibility for patients' care over a number of specialists, but does not detract from the idea that the patients must become intimately involved in their own care. Rather, this approach provides a consistent pool of information to the patient and the referring physician about the diagnosis, the etiology of the chronic "pain," and the rationale for the recommended, multifaceted therapy. This mutual understanding fosters the creation of more realistic attitudes about the ultimate success of treatment and puts the pain into a new perspective for patients and their physicians. Patients eventually realize that their chronic pain does not demand cessation of all social and occupational participation but rather imposes limitations on their activity and enjoyment of life, which are only as severe as they themselves choose.

Table 3–1. Reasons cited for avoiding the evaluation and treatment of patients with chronic pain

1. Doubt in practitioner's mind to believe the patient's suffering.
2. Lack of knowledge about "pain"—anatomy, pharmacology, the differences between acute and chronic pain.
3. Lack of time to devote to proper evaluation and management.
4. Long-term patient contact/care implied.
5. Whining, complaining, manipulative qualities of chronic pain patients.
6. Lack of enthusiasm to hear the same intractable complaints told in a long-winded fashion.
7. Unrevealing, nonconfirmatory laboratory results that make satisfactory diagnosis difficult.
8. Lack of ready availability of options for medical/surgical management.
9. Lack of completely successful treatment even in some well-handled cases.
10. Lack of support services in the medical community.
11. Frequent demands for paperwork input into the social system (legal, insurance, compensation).

WHAT IS PAIN?

Pain is a personal, subjective experience that is common in life. It can be associated with injury such as broken bones or muscle strains/sprains, diseases such as appendicitis or myocardial infarction, medical diagnostic/therapeutic procedures such as bone marrow biopsy or surgery, or emotional trauma such as the broken heart of love. It is the most common complaint of patients seeking medical care. As extrapolated by Bonica, it is estimated that annually 15 percent to 20 percent and 25 percent to 30 percent of people have acute and chronic pain problems respectively.[2, 3]

Pain means different things to different people and may have a different meaning to the same person under various circumstances. The individual episodes of pain have effects that far exceed the confines of the patient. As if the potential devastation of the individual's life is not significant enough, the cost to society due to pain evaluation, workup, treatment, missed workdays, and other expenses is great. The patient's pain impacts upon the immediate family as well as relatives, employers, fellow employees, community folk, and society.[2, 3]

Pain has recently been defined as "an unpleasant sensory and emotional experience associated with actual or potential tissue damage or described in terms of such damage."[4] This significant statement emphasizes that every pain, be it acute or chronic, is the result of a combination of physical and cognitive/affective factors. Understanding this and acknowledging it in practice is mandatory if one is to provide contemporary care to patients with pain. Furthermore, the patient who is having problems with pain must come to understand this concept as well. Even with a suitable definition of pain, there are other problems that contribute to pain's mismanagement and perpetuate its personal and societal impact (see table 3—2).

The significant differences between acute and chronic pain have become well established[2, 5] and are mentioned frequently in this textbook. Suffice it to say here, acute pain is a biologically necessary physiologic response that, through its function to notify the body of impending or ongoing tissue damage, triggers an escape reaction so that the damage will be diminished or even eliminated.[6] Nearly all experience episodes of acute pain during their lifetimes and become

Table 3–2. Problems of pain evaluation and management

1. In the past the definition of pain has varied according to the physician's specialty and orientation.
2. Current scientific, mathematical ways to measure and quantitate pain are inadequate.
3. Pain is a subjective, personal experience with only the patient's behavior as an outward, albeit inexact, sign.
4. Pain can have diverse meanings, can have different expressions, and can produce different reactions.
5. The amount of research in proportion to the magnitude of the problem is minimal, and there are poor experimental models, more so for chronic pain than for acute pain.
6. Research goes on in many different specialty areas, and the communication of discoveries and findings among the many different specialty groups is not well coordinated.
7. Little is taught about what is known, and, unfortunately, what is taught is poorly applied.

conditioned to the scenario of injury-sympathy-workup-treatment-relief from pain.

When the pain does not disappear after weeks to months of treatment, it is referred to as chronic pain.[2–4] Bonica states that chronic pain is arbitrarily defined as that which lasts longer than six months or beyond the normal course of the disease or injury.[6] The patient may have an obvious physical disease that is in part characterized by recurrent, intermittent episodes of pain such as cancer or low back pain, a continuous, progressive disease such as arthritis with which constant pain is usually associated, or chronic pain without a specific etiology, such as headaches or backaches. Whatever the cause, as pain endures the passage of time the patient faces frustration and despair in evaluation and treatment, repeated physical and emotional stress, and usually lifestyle disruption.[7,8]

Declaring the differences between acute and chronic pain is crucial because the extent of the workup and the treatment options considered are different, and the realistic possibilities of "cure" vary tremendously. One cannot simply apply the principles of acute pain treatment, at which most practitioners become proficient, to all pain. Treating all pain the same regardless of its etiology is not logical, nor will it reliably result in successful pain control.

Headaches and low back pain are chronic pain problems that account for the highest percentage of visits to physicians and formal pain centers.[9,10] Other patients are referred with cervical and/or shoulder pain, vascular/vasospastic disorders, pain related to cancer, and pain complaints for which no organic etiology has yet been identified. The referring physician must understand the services offered by the pain facility, as the scope of multidisciplinary involvement varies considerably among clinics.

THE DIAGNOSTIC STATE OF AFFAIRS

In spite of incredible advances in understanding about pain mechanisms, neuroanatomy, and neurophysiology[1, 11-16], the single biggest obstacle in pain evaluation is the lack of a method to quantitate these phenomena in the scientific and numerical modes we in medicine are so accustomed to. Although diaries, drawings, pain scales, and chemical assays have been proposed, we are still lacking a definitive, all-conclusive diagnostic test that can validate the presence, intensity, and severity of pain. There are diagnostic tests for some obvious physical injuries such as herniated discs or broken bones, but we still have no test that focuses on the patient's "reactions" to those pains. In fact, when one acknowledges the previously noted contemporary definition of pain, the expectation that a blood test or a chemical assay could effectively reflect the patient's pain is not fulfilled. We are left with techniques that assess the patient's behavioral reaction to pain, but these methods of quantitation are fraught with hazard and are highly unreliable.

There is pressure today, given the sophisticated equipment and advanced technology available, to overcome this diagnostic obstacle. Medical practice is strongly based on precise diagnosis and rapid cure. Thus, the failure to meet this expectation when chronic pain is managed is not well tolerated. The issue is magnified by data that reveal that up to 20 percent of patients with postoperative pain do not get effective analgesia[17], by the failure of many patients with pain secondary to cancer to get adequate pain relief[6, 18], and by the documented undertreatment of pain in hospitalized medical patients.[19-21] Moreover, the lack of a physical cause for pain does not necessarily implicate a psychological one[22].

Given the lack of accurate diagnostic testing, the practitioner is left with the classic sources of information: history-taking, physical examination, and laboratory assessment. Each area of investigation has a contribution to make in the patient's evaluation. The patient must be given an opportunity to tell *his* story *his* way. The implied investment in time associated with this approach may discourage some from interacting with such patients, but the critical information revealed—from what's told and how it's told—is necessary to the thorough evaluation of the patient. Since most complaints of pain have a vast differential diagnosis, the practitioner must systematically review the patient. Yet the evaluation process must be streamlined when possible via efficient documented evaluation tools and protocols to neither delay treatment nor unnecessarily extend the patient's suffering.

The historical review of the patient must include a characterization of the pain. Crucial to the review is elucidating when and where the pain began and under what circumstances, how the pain is described (sharp, stabbing, burning, aching), what makes it better and worse, what other symptoms are associated with it, and what it truly prevents the patient from doing.

Closely allied with the history of the pain is the treatment history. One is interested in noting which modalities have already been tried and how the patient rates their success. A statement of the patient's current daily treatment program is also vital, as is an assessment of the patient's compliance with the recommended treatment. The pain, treatment, and general medical histories should be obtained from all patients, whether their pain is acute or chronic. One must decipher whether the current pain episode is a "typical" one or may herald the onset of new problems.

In patients whose pain complaints have become chronic in nature, attention *must be* directed to factors that can modify the presentation of pain. The consequences of the pain on the patient's life *must* be analyzed. Aspects of the patient's occupational, social and psychological histories must be investigated, as listed in table 3–3 and 3–4. Though the patient may be able to tolerate the physical pain, the impact of the "pain" on the patient's family, lifestyle, marriage, or work attendance may result in intolerable circumstances. Treatment planning will be extremely difficult until the pain's true operative mechanisms are elucidated and considered. The patient's personal opinion about the meaning of the pain must also be solicited, acknowledged, and dealt with. This information is a crucial part of the data base upon which treatment will ultimately be predicated.

The physical examination correlates the pain complaints with anatomic possibilities and generally sorts out pathology of the innumerable body structures that could cause the pain. The appropriate physical examination will depend upon

Table 3–3. Pain evaluation: issues in the occupational history

1.	Physical and mental/educational status of the patient
2.	Physical and intellectual demands of the current job
3.	Duration of current employment
4.	Employment goals/desires
5.	Satisfaction with job
6.	Employer/employee relationship

Table 3–4. Pain evaluation: issues in the social history

1.	Family composition
2.	Impact of the patient's inability to work
3.	Current income status
4.	Marital status
5.	Spouse's work situation
6.	Community resources for retraining or alternate employment opportunities
7.	Family history of disabling illness
8.	Desire for social, recreational, sexual activity

the patient's unique pain problem and the evaluator's interest and available time. It is important to have physical data in the patient's record for comparison to past examinations and the documentation of improvement as treatment ensues. Patients with chronic pain can develop progressive pathology, and all pain is not necessarily explained by or related to their chronic pain problem. If there are questions or suspect findings, a specialty referral is advisable because the sooner the pain is thoroughly evaluated and all questions answered, the sooner the patient will be presented with an accurate status statement and appropriate therapy initiated.

Physical assessment may involve inspection of the patient; auscultation of the chest, abdomen, or vascular structures; palpation; and neurosensory examination. Areas of sensory deficit must be identified as must motor weakness and reflex asymmetry. Range of motion of involved joints (flexion, extension, rotation) is important as is a functional assessment of related musculoskeletal structures. Areas of muscle spasm must be located and myofascial trigger points marked. The patient must be observed while lying down, sitting, walking, bending, and changing position. Lengths of the arms or legs may be important as may circumference measurements in muscular or swollen areas. The vascular status of the extremities should be noted with the usual means, and skin temperature measurements may offer valuable data.

The third major area of patient data is laboratory test results. It is fundamental that we acknowledge the lack of a diagnostic test for every conceivable cause of pain. In considering laboratory testing, one wants to prevent the needless duplication of expensive tests and unnecessary discomfort by obtaining only those that will truly affect the way a given patient is treated or referred. As the sophistication of one's pain practice increases, it is likely that access to and a tendency to order more tests will be manifest. Actually, this may be an implied expectation in the referral of a patient. As with physical examinations, some laboratory tests performed in serial fashion will help to document treatment response.

It is crucial that all consultants guard against the erroneous and fruitless conclusion that negative laboratory tests mean that patients have no real pain and their "pains" must be all in their heads. This conclusion is entirely nonproductive and likely to provoke patients to prove their pain through more aggressive, adverse behavioral means.

THE ROLE OF PSYCHOLOGICAL SERVICES IN THE EVALUATION OF CHRONIC PAIN

Since the inception of the multidisciplinary pain clinic model in the mid-1960s, psychological services have contributed significantly to patient care and are integrated with the other disciplines represented in the clinic setting. In the typical multidisciplinary pain clinic, the psychological evaluation process combines both clinical assessment methods, often in the form of an interview, which will be described in some detail later in this section, and formal measurement. For purposes of discussion, formal measurement techniques employed in the pain clinic setting may be divided into screening inventories, which are data base packages that often include pain self-reports, psychological assessment techniques, and behavioral and psychophysical assessment methods. The data gleaned from the evaluation process assist in making decisions about intervention approaches.

Screening inventories

A major decision for any pain clinic is the form of the data base package to be administered to all patients. In addition to serving obvious clinical needs regarding the presenting pain problem, generating an appropriate data base assists in developing research questions and allows follow-up evaluation of treatment effectiveness.

A number of screening inventories have been described[23,24], and some are formatted for easy computer storage and data retrieval.[25] Although the contents of the inventories vary, most include basic demographic questions, items related to interference of pain with basic life functions, and factors influencing pain relief or exacerbation. In addition many clinics include in their assessment packages some type of self-report pain measure. Examples of this would be a visual analogue (linear) scale on which patients indicate their current level of experienced pain[26], the McGill Pain Questionnaire[27], which requires a choice of adjectival descriptors of pain, or the use of pain maps or drawings.[28]

The psychologist in the pain clinic setting may wish to include some more traditional evaluation techniques that provide direct information on emotional functioning. Instruments such as the MMPI (Minnesota Multiphasic Personality Inventory) or the SCL-90 (Symptom Checklist-90)[29], initially developed and employed with psychiatric population, are now frequently used to assess chronic pain patients. Although most patients may not require an extensive, traditional psychological workup, a brief inventory can provide valuable information on the extent of depression and anxiety and the likelihood that emotional factors or life stressors will amplify somatic complaints. Examples of such inventories include the Zung Depression Inventory[30], the Taylor Manifest Anxiety Scale[31], or the Social Readjustment Rating Scale.[32] In addition, more specialized psychological instruments have been designed specifically for chronic pain populations[33, 34] or subpopulations such as chronic headache[35] or chronic temporomandibular joint dysfunction.[36] Generally, the latter class of instruments will be most beneficial to the independent practitioner who needs assistance in referring patients with pain to more specialized settings. The psychologist will usually have a preference regarding the assessment methods employed, but the basic concept underlying any of these methods is to provide a standardized set of conditions for obtaining data and to compare such data with available norms or base rates in the population.

The clinical interview

The clinical interview is usually the initial contact between the patient and the psychologist in the multidisciplinary pain clinic setting. Although often minimally prepared through written materials from the pain clinic or information provided by the referring clinician, the patient brings to the interview preconceptions based on popularized notions of psychologists or psychiatrists or predicated on previous contacts with mental health professionals not trained in chronic pain management. For this reason it is helpful to provide some initial explanation and reassurances about the psychologist's role on the pain clinic team. For example, it is important to assure the patient at the outset of the interview that contact with the psychologist neither impugns the reality of pain nor implies a mental disturbance. Instead, the psychologist may facilitate understanding the impact of chronic pain on vocational roles and personal relationships and eventually assist the patient in *coping* with pain.

The direction of the interview generally proceeds from the somatic to the psychological. Because pain and physical distress are the presenting issues, the patient may be asked to describe circumstances associated with pain onset, the nature and utility of prior interventions, and changes in the frequency, intensity, or quality of the pain over time. In this process, information is gathered about potential conflictual circumstances surrounding the pain problem (e.g., anger with a work supervisor, traumatic injury with resultant fear of returning to the site of injury), the degree to which pain complaints and symptoms have been reinforced by prior health care providers and relatives, and the patient's belief system regarding possibilities for altering pain by self or others.

The conclusion of the pain history is a convenient time to assess depression, a frequent concomitant of chronic pain. Although pain patients frequently deny feeling depressed, they quite often will acknowledge biological or vegetative depressive symptoms. These include insomnia, classically early morning awakening, lowered energy, appetite and weight loss, lowered libido, and frequently passive and even active suicidal ideation. These symptoms are often frightening and alien to the patient's usual emotional state. It is helpful to provide some assurances that such symptoms often accompany chronic pain and are likely to resolve as treatment progresses. If depressive symptoms *preceded* or occurred concurrently with the onset of pain, a major depressive disorder may be etiologically significant. In these cases, treating the depression frequently produces significant pain relief.[37]

The next phase of the interview centers on assessing how the pain affects significant areas of life functioning, including work, avocational interests, and spousal and other interpersonal relationships. Important questions here include how the patient spends time during the day. Is significant time spent reclining and avoiding previously enjoyed activities? Is the behavioral style one of compulsively overworking on a day when the pain is improved and remaining in bed on subsequent days because of difficulties in self-pacing? How does the patient interact with the spouse and significant others with regard to pain? In general, what does the pain allow the patient to gain and avoid, and what other current sources of satisfaction exist in the patient's life? One important question that should always be included in the interview relates to past or current physical or sexual abuse. A recent survey revealed that 53 percent of 153 women who presented to a hospital-based chronic pain center reported a previous history of sexual or physical abuse, and in all cases the pain followed the abusive episodes.[38]

Finally, it is useful in the interview to learn about the patient's developmental and past medical history. Topics of particular interest include prior exposure to pain models, childhood illness history and behavioral responses to past illnesses, school or interpersonal problems during childhood and adolescence, and a history of physically or emotionally abusive relationships with parents and caretakers.

Behavioral and physiological assessment

In addition to the more generic information provided by self-report pain measures and the clinical interview, behavioral and physiological assessment methods focus on more specific, directly observable responses associated with pain. These include time spent out of bed (uptime), grimacing, complaints of pain, medication use, degree of attention from significant others, and level of muscular and autonomic activity under differing conditions. The utility of behavioral methods is underscored by reports suggesting low correlations between pain description and level of activity[39] or organic impairment.[40] However, behavioral and physiological data may be integrated within a broader assessment package that respects the complexity of the clinical pain phenomenon.

Two general strategies for behaviorally assessing chronic pain employ observation and automatic recording devices. In self-observation, the patient may be asked to record hourly in a diary the amount of time spent reclining, upright, and walking.[41] This can be transformed into graphic data at appropriate intervals to provide a visual chart of patient progress. Another type of behavioral observation is to videotape or time-sample patient behavior and rate specific categories related to pain display. A recently developed grading system for pain behaviors[42] is reported to yield valid and reliable ratings of motor behaviors, including guarded movement, bracing, rubbing, grimacing, and sighing. In addition, rating scales appropriate for ward observation by nurses[43] or for assessing pain behaviors in an interview setting[44] have been described.

An important potential source of reinforcement for pain behavior is the spouse, who should be included in at least part of the interview. In a recent finding that suggests the connection of spousal relationship issues and pain, couples with a high degree of marital satisfaction evidenced higher levels of physiological reactivity when the patient displayed pain behaviors. In couples with low marital satisfaction no differential reactivity was found.[45]

Automatic recording devices eliminate some biases of the observational method but are limited to motor behaviors. One example is a highly reliable and valid automatic recording device developed by Sanders[46] that contains a mercury-tilt switch for measuring uptime. An interesting finding is that very low correlations were obtained among instrument recordings, self-observation, and other observational ratings of time spent upright.[47]

Another assessment role frequently provided by the psychologist in the pain clinic relates to the evaluation of physiological response systems. This may range from obtaining baseline EMG levels before biofeedback treatment to multimodally assessing autonomic responses under conditions of stress and relaxation. In spite of increasing mechanical sophistication in physiological measurement devices, the research literature has been quite inconsistent regarding physiological responses unique to chronic pain. For example, low back pain patients do not differ from pain-free controls on levels of EMG activity in back muscles under conditions of either stress or relaxation.[48] Neither do low back pain patients demonstrate different autonomic arousal patterns (e.g., heart rate, skin conductance) than pain-free controls.[49] A more promising direction in physiological assessment relates to patterns, rather than to absolute levels, of muscle activity in chronic pain patients. Some initial research has indicated asymmetrical activity when the EMG of muscles of the left and right sides of the back are compared in patients with low back pain.[50] Other studies[51] have suggested that postural factors such as prolonged standing accentuate asymmetrical muscle activity and argue for bilateral assessment under differing patterns of activity.

This discussion serves to illustrate some of the evaluative functions provided by the psychologist in the pain clinic setting. Furthermore, as most psychologists tend to identify with the scientist-practitioner professional model, the assessment process frequently generates and is modified by research findings. Thus, a distinctive contribution of the psychologist, one that can benefit all members of the treatment team, is the close alignment of clinical and research skills.

EVALUATION—SUMMARY

The evaluation scheme for the patient with chronic pain must establish the diagnosis for the patient's complaints. In this era, the comprehensive diagnosis demanded takes into account the physical and the nonphysical contributions to

Table 3–5. Outline of evaluation and treatment methods for chronic pain

A. Evaluation
   1. Static information
      (a). pain history
      (b). treatment, past and current
      (c). general medical history
      (d). occupational history
      (e). psychosocial status screening inventories, interview behavioral and physiological assessment
      (f). the patient's perception of pain
   2. Physical assessment
      (a). neurologic
      (b). orthopedic
      (c). functional
   3. Laboratory diagnosis

B. Management
   1. medications—narcotics, nonnarcotics, detoxification, adjunctive drugs
   2. Surgery—definitive, palliative, neuro-ablative
   3. Nerve blocks—local anesthetic drugs, steroids, neurolytic agents, narcotics
   4. Stimulation techniques—TENS, acupuncture
   5. Physical rehabilitation—exercise, orthotics, formal therapy
   6. Psychotherapeutics—biofeedback, relaxation training, hypnosis, self-regulation techniques
   7. Rehabilitation—activity restoration, social reentry, vocational, psychological

the pain. Only by achieving this complete understanding of the patient will therapy that addresses *the many needs of the patient* be recommended. By clarifying the significance of the "pain" to the patient, one will more fully appreciate the extraneous factors that are modifying the patient's complaints and behavior. Table 3–5 summarizes the evaluation protocol and outlines the therapeutic techniques to be discussed. No patient is denied the benefit of treatment planning. However, realistic expectations for the results of therapy must be engendered in both the patient and the health care professionals by considering these data in reference to a patient.

The information garnered by the psychologist in the evaluative setting must be shared with the members of the multidisciplinary staff. This may be done in timely meetings attended by all pain clinic professionals. The advantage of this approach is that psychological data can be integrated into the overall treatment plan and may be useful in addressing issues such as compliance, motivation for improvement, or even choice of somatic intervention. Likewise, information obtained from professionals evaluating the physiological components of the pain problem may be important in structuring components of the psychological-behavioral intervention.

CONSIDERATIONS IN TREATMENT OF PATIENTS WITH PAIN PROBLEMS

Patients bring to the clinical setting their experiences of successful treatment for acute pain problems. Everyone expects that broken bones can be successfully treated with casts, and many operations for painful conditions such as appendicitis

Table 3–6. Treatment goals in chronic pain using the multidisciplinary approach

1.	Decrease the frequency and intensity of the patient's pain. In some patients, eliminate pain.
2.	Decrease the need for and use of potent medications.
3.	Avoid unnecessary surgery.
4.	Increase the patient's insight into physical pain and the nonphysical influences thereon.
5.	Enhance the patient's abilities to cope with residual pain.
6.	Increase the patient's functional capabilities in spite of residual pain.

and cholecystitis are routinely successful. It is a matter of philosophy whether the pathophysiologic consequences of acute pain are what demand treatment or whether it is primarily the anguish and suffering that the patient wants relieved.

When the patient is confronted with chronic pain, a high degree of suffering and frustration may result from the lack of complete treatment success an expectation contrary to the patient's past experiences. Thus, it is important that the patient understand the realistic goals for treatment of chronic pain (see table 3–6). These goals stress coping and pain control not necessarily elimination, although it is not excluded. They are aimed at decreasing utilization of the health care system by patients with chronic problems, restoring the patient to a more functional and productive activity level, and normalizing the home and social environment.[52]

The treatment options for chronic pain are based upon understanding the significant differences between acute and chronic pain. Basically, many of the modalities so successfully applied in the management of acute pain problems cannot be applied with similar success in the *long-term* management of chronic pain patients. The patient deserves an explanation of the diagnosis and the rationale for the treatment options chosen. The fundamental concept of the treatment program is that each alternative employed will result in a certain percentage decrease in the patient's pain. Thus, while any single modality taken alone may provide a decrease of only 10 percent or 20 percent in the patient's complaints, when two or three such options are used in a coordinated program, the total decrease in the patient's pain will be significant. Without this understanding the patient will see the use of many of the same treatments that had been applied in the past in singular fashion as nothing more than the doctor's lack of understanding about the severity of the pain and as diminishing the significance of the pain problem.

In general, the patient should be presented with the concept that pain can be significantly reduced and perhaps eliminated by the use of medications, surgery, nerve blocks, and counterstimulation techniques (TENS, acupuncture).[53] The decrease in pain should permit an increase in the patient's activity level. For patients with an acute pain problem, that activity level will likely be their normal routine. For patients with chronic pain, that activity level will not likely be the normal routine but rather some portion of it. For specific positive feedback about activity freedom and progress, patients can engage in exercise programs. This physical therapy approach will additionally benefit by helping reverse the detrimental consequences of prolonged restricted activity or self-imposed inactivity.

As the pain declines and confidence in physical capabilities is restored, the patient faces the reality that some of the chronic pain will not be so easy to eliminate. Any patient deserves encouragement and support to remain compliant with treatment and enthusiastic about progress. A select number may benefit further from formal psychotherapeutic intervention to bolster their ability to cope with residual pain. The ultimate goal of treatment is complete rehabilitation to the patient's former productive lifestyle and occupational pursuits. In chronic pain management this ideal frequently is not achievable, yet satisfactory activity levels can frequently be restored and social reintegration accomplished.

PHARMACOLOGIC MANAGEMENT

The convenience, simplicity, innumerable variety, and ready availability of medications frequently make them a first choice for the treatment of many medical conditions. In pain management it is significant that many practitioners believe that analgesics can be prescribed before the pain has been explained, and patients encourage this approach with a "take-a-pill" philosophy. The generic use of analgesic medications is perceived as reasonable because many patients with chronic, ongoing pain problems have had unrevealing workups and are left with only the nonspecific complaint of pain. Analgesic medications are then prescribed in a manner routine to the physician. Unfortunately, this naive approach does not necessarily correlate with the known pharmacokinetics and pharmacodynamics of the medications, the suspected mechanism for the pain, or the use of a drug appropriate for the severity of the pain.[54–56] Even the significant differences between the anti-inflammatory action of aspirin and acetaminophen may be forgotten.

As the medications so useful in treating acute pain are continued in the management of chronic pain, a tolerance to the desired effect of the medication develops. Usually this necessitates an increased dosage of medication which may be repeated over the course of a number of visits to the physician while the patient continues to complain of pain. Ultimately, this approach can contribute to the patient's overuse and/or misuse of the medication. Frequently, a point is reached after which further increases in dosage contribute only to undesirable, detrimental side effects.[57] Then the patient may seek the advice of any number of physicians for a growing number of symptoms and drug-related side effects that are not adequately managed by the prescribed therapy. This puts the patients at risk for taking a number of medications that when viewed in toto would reveal that illogical, ineffective combinations are being emloyed.

Frequently, patients with chronic pain seem to be passively overtreated with medications.[58–59] The pharmacologic profile may become compounded by the open or occult use of alcohol, which enhances the chemical depression associated with the potent analgesics and sedative/hypnotic drugs frequently prescribed. These induced changes alter patients' cognitive and perceptual abilities to react to and cope with environmental stressors relative to their pain.[60]

Upon referral, oftentimes, a patient has been taking a myriad of drugs for weeks to months, the pain has persisted in spite of the concoction of pharmacologic agents prescribed, and side effects are the only manifestation of any drug use. Thus, the patient cannot ignore or object to the logic of withdrawing these medications.[61] Any patient who fails to understand the importance of this step ought to raise the specialist's suspicion that drug-seeking behavior is perhaps a dominant goal of the patient. The details of drug detoxification are beyond the scope of this discussion. Suffice it to say, most medications can be gradually withdrawn by decreasing the daily dose by 10 percent every three to four days and providing, if clinically necessary, concurrent medications that treat some of the expected side effects of withdrawal.

In the outpatient setting it is desirable to provide the patient with a day-by-day, dose-by-dose, drug-by-drug, handwritten schedule for detoxification. This gives the patient a very systematic way to decrease the doses of the innumerable medications that may be taken and thereby minimizes the potential for annoying withdrawal side effects. It is entirely possible that some patients will need to be admitted to a hospital setting for more controlled detoxification from high-dose narcotics, barbiturate drugs, or unspecified multidrug use.

The goal of detoxification is to eventually have the patients using medications that are more benign when taken on a chronic basis than are many of the narcotic and sedative/hypnotic/tranquilizer drugs. This concept becomes even more reasonable when other therapeutic modalities are also recommended and employed.[52] The basal analgesia provided by drugs such as acetaminophen and the nonsteroidal anti-inflammatory drugs (NSAIDs)[57,62–65] can be potentiated by the use of adjunctive medications, such as the tricyclic antidepressants[66–69] and the phenothiazines.[70-72] These combinations are prescribed with the full knowledge that by themselves they may not significantly decrease the patient's pain. But, as one component of a total treatment program, their contribution to the decrease of pain will achieve significance.[56,73]

The physician must be prepared to defend this apparent demotion in the potency of medications to the patient, referring doctors, and perhaps lawyers and insurance companies. The decrease in the potency of medications does not downplay the severity of the pain. Rather, it is based upon the desire to achieve partial pain control with medications that will have few side effects when used on a long-term basis. These principles should be applied to all pain patients, even those with cancer.[74] When the daily level of pain acutely changes, all the prescribing physician's pharmacological knowledge and pain management skill must be used to treat the patient effectively yet safely with the potent drugs available.[55,74,75]

There certainly is a need for more education about the pharmacokinetics and pharmacodynamics of all drugs used in pain management so that they can be applied in a more scientific and beneficial fashion. In the future, medication application may involve the use of transdermal drugs and drugs that can be applied in a sublingual fashion. Also, combinations of the NSAIDs with certain narcotic agonist/

antagonist drugs may provide more versatility in pharmacologic practice. The application of patient-controlled analgesia (PCA) systems is a modernistic technology to provide a patient with pain relief in a simple, adaptable manner. PCA allows a patient to self-administer a preset dose of narcotic intravenously while the programmable device provides a subsequent lockout period during which no further drug can be delivered. [76–70] Experience with these techniques must first be gained in clinically controlled environments, such as in the management of postoperative pain and patients with pain related to cancer. Eventually they will be used by selected patients with nonmalignant chronic pain.

SURGERY

Surgical intervention in the management of pain is as much an option as any other therapeutic modality. The fact that surgical intervention is invasive and has associated morbidity and mortality dictates its use for only specific indications and with realistic expectations at both ends of the scalpel. Many definitive surgical procedures, when directed at specific, identifiable pathology, are highly successful. The hazards of the surgery and the necessary anesthetic must be weighed against the realistic potential for benefit from the procedure. Intractable pain can develop after surgery[13,79], when adhesions or neuromas in the surgical area become pain generators.

It is now well recognized from years of experience that surgical procedures aimed at simply transecting the nervous system to disrupt the transmission of pain impulses do not necessarily result in long-term pain relief.[80,81] New appreciation for the fact that the transmission of pain impulses to the central nervous system is not confined to a single neural network helps one to understand this result. There are a number of sensory input and modulatory systems. Thus, a simple transectional procedure cannot guarantee a permanent bypass of the complex neural anatomy involved. Destructive neurosurgical procedures are frequently considered only in patients with pain secondary to malignancy and when the patient's life expectancy is perceived to be consistent with the expected duration of pain relief but not with the onset of miserable side effects.

The recent elaboration of the concept of plasticity also helps us to understand why destructive neurosurgical procedures and even neurolytic blocks do not provide long-term relief.[14–16] Plasticity is one of the body's mechanisms for attempting to overcome the consequences of disruption of the neural system. This repair process can potentially contribute to a chronic pain syndrome. Further, it is likely that this reparative process will not restore all the usual inhibitory and facilitory controls on sensory input. Therefore, impulse transmission through areas subject to neural repair may gain unimpeded access to higher brain centers where the phenomenon of pain is determined.[13]

Lastly, there is new appreciation for the neuroanatomy of pain entry circuits in the nervous system. Fifteen to twenty percent of sensory input to the nervous system may come through the anterior spinal nerve root.[8,82] This is significant because procedures to interrupt sensory input that are aimed solely at the dorsal root entry zone (so called DREZ lesions) cannot be expected to provide total sensory elimination. Thus, patients who undergo dorsal root rhizotomies and who complain of returning pain can at least be provided an explanation as to why the surgical procedure did not totally eliminate pain. They may also be given insight into the complexity of the pain problem now that healed areas of the nervous system may be contributing to the continuing pain problem.

In the future, fewer destructive neurosurgical procedures may be done and better surgical techniques may be utilized in all pain management surgery. Examples of this would include microsurgical techniques for operating on herniated discs and percutaneous, selective nerve manipulation procedures. The use of lasers for surgery and focal injection/stereotactic procedures (radiofrequency neurolysis, cryoanalgesia) may become better developed.

NERVE BLOCKS

Certainly, the most common intervention provided by anesthesiologists in the management of pain patients is the application of regional anesthetic techniques for diagnostic and/or therapeutic purposes.[10] In the grand scheme of pain control, nerve blocks are but one component of a total treatment program.[83] Yet, by providing prompt, temporary relief with local anesthetic drugs, occasionally in combination with steroids (when nerve inflammation is thought to be part of the pain's etiology), significant diminution of the patient's pain can be accomplished. This has the subsequent benefits of decreasing the need for potent medications or surgery, enhancing the patient's attitude about reachieving health, and encouraging a positive attitude about cooperating with other components of therapy. Thus, nerve blocks alone can be a very potent intervention and should be considered readily in the management of patients with pain. The advantages of nerve blocks are that they are nonaddictive, can be repeated frequently, may be performed on an outpatient basis, generally have few side effects as compared to medications and surgery, and involve interaction with the patient.

To balance the discussion, there are risks to the patient receiving nerve block therapy because of the invasive nature of the procedure. Complications can result from the drug injected or the technique itself. The technical skill of the anesthesiologist may have a bearing on the incidence of failure, especially for the more complicated or uncommon nerve blocks. However, regional anesthetic techniques for pain control are becoming a more common component of the general practice of anesthesiology.

Thus the techniques, their clinical applications, and the subsequent management of patients if complications do arise will be increasingly familiar to more anesthesiologists. It is then only a matter of using discretion to select appropriate patients and choosing the optimal time to intervene with this most potent therapy. As stressed before, one must always have a specific diagnosis for which the procedures are being done and at least enough workup to identify the usual contraindications to regional anesthesia.

A number of specific nerve blocks can be used in the management of common pain syndromes. Differential nerve blocks (i.e., subarachnoid or epidural techniques) are advocated in selected patients when the etiology of the pain complaints is obscure.[84, 85] If the inciting pathology for pain can be localized to the sympathetic, somatosensory, motor, or higher CNS systems, more precise nerve block techniques can be used in the ongoing management of the patient.

Some regional anesthetic procedures used for operative anesthesia can be continued into the postoperative period to provide very effective control of pain. These techniques include the use of local anesthetic drugs[86–89] which, because of their relatively short duration of action, must be administered by intermittent injection or infusion devices, and the exciting new use of traditional narcotic drugs with perispinal techniques.[90–92] While the use of local anesthetic drugs results in residual sensory and sympathetic block (proportional to the concentration of the local anesthetic used), perispinal narcotics provide potent analgesia without interruption of other neurologic function. However, the variable occurrence of side effects, such as itching, nausea, vomiting, urinary retention, and delayed respiratory depression, must be dealt with.

An extensive literature documents the efficacy of epidural blocks with local anesthetic and steroids in the management of radicular low back pain[93, 94], sympathetic nervous system blocks in reflex sympathetic dystrophy and causalgia[95–98], and various nerve blocks in cancer pain control.[99, 100] The application of neurolytic blocks using alcohol or phenol truly represents the ultimate in rapport between doctor and patient and requires understanding the goals of treatment and impeccable technical skill. Nerve blocks performed with neurolytic agents have a definite place in the management of selected patients, but these techniques are primarily applied to those with pain secondary to malignancy.[99, 100]

In the future, greater understanding is needed as to why techniques such as the intravenous infusion of local anesthetics (lidocaine) can result in pain relief.[101] We also need to better understand why the use of local anesthetic drugs alone can frequently result in pain relief that lasts weeks to months, well beyond the expected pharmacologic duration of action of the drug injected. Hopefully, pain center programs will more clearly define the precise role for nerve blocks in pain management and investigate the use of alternate drugs for injection therapy. Certainly, the more widespread use of perispinal narcotics in selected groups of patients will require the continuing intervention of anesthesiologists in pain control.

STIMULATION TECHNIQUES

That hyperstimulation of the nervous system using large, nonpain fibers could drown out pain signals that travel in small, pain-transmitting fibers was the basic premise of the Gate Control Theory presented by Melzack and Wall in 1965[1] and was modified in later years by the same investigators.[11, 12] We have all used this pain-reduction method before. Common examples would be pinching your finger in the door or being kicked in the shin and reacting by sucking the wounded digit or rubbing the damaged shin. The physical action of sucking your finger or rubbing the shin activates large-fiber input to the nervous system, and seems to diminish the original pain. Early clinical therapeutic attempts to provide hyperstimulation using electrodes placed in the epidural space or implanted in the substance of the dorsal column of the spinal cord did not result in consistently high rates of success and are currently of only limited availability in a few medical centers around the country.[102]

Acupuncture is an ancient technique that has usefulness in the management of pain but has not been demonstrated satisfactorily to provide consistent pain relief to a great majority of patients.[103, 104] It is likely that with more research in this field some form of this technique will regain clinical significance in the future. Currently, acupuncture is limited clinically by variable licensure requirements for practitioners, the need for special therapists, poor documentation of positive effect, and indifferent third-party reimbursement for such therapy.

Clinically, the most practical form of hyperstimulation of the nervous system is transcutaneous electrical nerve stimulation (TENS).[102] The formal technique involves the use of battery-powered pulse generators, the output of which can be set by the therapist and controlled by the patient. TENS stimulates large-fiber input to a gating mechanism in the substantia gelatinosa area of the dorsal horn of the spinal cord and may activate the endorphin system. This input modifies incoming pain messages traveling along small, pain-transmitting fibers. The stimulation is provided on contact with the skin of carbonized rubber electrodes that can be placed over traditional acupuncture points, over blood vessels to stimulate sympathetic fibers, or over the dermatomal distribution of peripheral nerves.

TENS units have been effectively applied in the treatment of acute sport injuries[102, 105], chronic pain problems[102, 105], postoperative pain[105–107], and specific problems ranging from the treatment of bladder spasm and pain[108] to the treatment of severe angina.[109] The prime advantages of TENS are that it is noninvasive and patient-controlled. Further, it is simple enough to teach patients so that a special therapist is not continually needed, portable enough to be used anywhere, free of major systemic side effects (so it does not interfere with the patient's other desired activities or treatment modalities), not age-restricted, and uses some of the body's own mechanisms for modulating pain input.

Though the technique has gained wide application, further research is needed to detail the specific pathologic conditions for which it is most effective and to clarify the frequencies and intensity of stimulation and amplitude control for specific problems. Because TENS has been so generically applied, some do not perceive it to be so effective. But when a conscious decision is made to use it as a component in the overall treatment program for properly selected patients, a significant degree of pain reduction can be achieved.

PHYSICAL REHABILITATION

As pain is reduced through the judicious use of medications, surgery, nerve blocks, and stimulation techniques, the patient must translate the decrease in pain into an increase in function and activity. If this does not occur over a reasonable period of time, the validity of the primary diagnosis may be questioned. It is possible that just decreasing or even eliminating the patient's pain does not immediately answer all of the many problems that are encountered by the patient with chronic pain.

Many of the pathophysiologic consequences of pain, for example, those associated with acute pain and its treatment (hypertension, tachycardia, anxiety, nausea, vomiting, urinary retention)[110], do not linger into the period of chronic pain. Rather, the patient suffers from a decrease in muscle tone and strength, a reduction in the range of motion of major joints, postural limitations, a decrease in energy and enthusiasm, a perceived growing intolerance to all physical activity, weight gain, and the appearance of nonproductive emotions such as frustration, hopelessness, and hostility. This desperate physical and emotional state must be reversed. Frequently, it can be documented by obtaining a history from the patient, if not the spouse, that a prolonged period of weeks' to months' duration has passed since the time of the original injury and that during this interval the patient has maintained a very low activity profile. If the patient's pain persists but the workup fails to reveal that the ongoing pain indicates ongoing tissue damage, the patient should be introduced to the logical concept that gradual, guided, rehabilitative physical programs can reverse the detrimental physical consequences of prolonged inactivity. As with the recommendations for medication change following failure to improve, the logical recommendation to increase activity should not meet with patient objections. It has been documented by Fordyce et al.[111] and Linton[112] that there is no correlation between the patient's complaints of chronic pain and performance of prescribed exercises and physical activity.

It is possible that many patients who complain of musculoskeletal pain will require formal physical therapy instruction for a limited period of time.[113,114] There must be an understanding that *formal* physical therapy will be time-limited because it is not in itself the significant activity. Rather, it is the patient's independent home activities after completion of the formal technique demonstrations that will ultimately determine the success of physical rehabilitation.[115] The challenge to develop self-help attitudes toward performing physical therapy is thoroughly consistent with the philosophy of chronic pain management. It is likely that the response to physical rehabilitation demands will provide an early indication of the patient's true motivation to improve and overall behavioral flexibility. Physical therapy and occupational and recreational programs must emphasize increasing range of motion and strength and restoring endurance for the patient in such activities as sitting, standing, and walking, let alone more aggressive, work-related activities.

PSYCHOLOGICAL THERAPEUTICS

As pain decreases and function increases, the patient will face the reality that not all the chronic pain can be eliminated. It is at this time that reinforcement, encouragement, and support will be needed. This sort of superficial psychotherapy can be provided by any caring and compassionate health care provider.[116, 117] Occasionally, there are patients in whom specific nonphysical contributions to the pain are more adequately managed by a specialist. There are a number of psychological techniques with therapeutic benefit in the management of chronic pain patients. However, consulting and referring physicians must not conclude from the lack of positive physical findings that the patient is suffering primarily from psychogenic pain or a stress reaction.[22]

Psychological interventions for chronic pain may be generally classified as coping strategies or environmental control techniques. Although these approaches must be interwoven with those of other specialists in the multidisciplinary setting, several general assumptions underlying psychological/behavioral strategies may enhance the outcomes of interventions from other professionals:

1. Techniques proposed by the psychologist are not likely to *cure* the pain but are more likely to significantly help the patient to live and *cope* with pain.
2. The patient has the capacity and the responsibility to exercise some control over the pain.
3. Chronic pain affects and is affected by factors external to the patient and the somatic symptoms.

Thus, the patient is aided in reframing expectations that pain will be abolished by a single procedure such as a nerve block or surgery. Furthermore, the patient is encouraged to focus on improvement in functioning rather than the previously frustrating experience of searching for etiologic factors to explain the basis of the pain.

Coping strategies for pain management

A number of techniques employed in pain clinic settings emphasize self-management or coping approaches. Some of these strategies are purported to have direct physiologic effects on causes of pain, for example, EMG biofeedback for low back pain[118] or temperature biofeedback for vascular headache.[119] However, more recent research[48, 120, 121] suggests that both relaxation training and biofeedback, which are frequently employed pain interventions, may have their effects primarily on an anxiolytic basis. Thus, psychological services make a major contribution by training patients in stress management.

Stress management approaches encourage the patient to develop coping responses when experiencing pain or pain-related stimuli such as anxiety or depressive cognitions. One set of these techniques is directed at altering physiological patterns associated with tension and anxiety and has the general effect of lowering autonomic arousal. Included here are procedures such as progressive muscle relaxation; deep breathing techniques; various biofeedback strategies designed to provide information on such physiological functioning parameters as muscle activity, peripheral vasodilation, heart rate, and blood pressure; and, aerobic exercise. Another set of procedures useful in coping skills training is aimed directly at cognitive factors associated with pain and discomfort. These include imagery and meditative approaches described by some authors in the context of hypnosis[122], as well as strategies of distraction or reinterpretation of painful stimuli.[44, 123] An interesting elaboration of this approach is provided by the cognitive-behavioral management techniques described by Meichenbaum and his colleagues.[124] These involve training in self-coaching and self-reinforcement for coping with stimuli associated with pain and anxiety.

Environmental control techniques

In contrast to training in coping strategies, which focuses on self-management of pain by generating alternative responses, environmental techniques are directed at altering the pain behaviors or factors that reinforce or maintain those behaviors in the patient's environment. Data from the interview or from the more formal self-report or behavioral assessment techniques mentioned earlier can guide environmental management approaches. In practice, three general categories of behavior are particularly important in the environmental control of chronic pain: (1) behaviors connected with the health care system, (2) attentional behaviors connected with the spouse and family members, (3) and avoidance behaviors by the patient connected with motor and purposeful activities. The psychologist can often help recommend effective behavior change in these three areas.

Although more detailed descriptions of behaviorally based programs that address environmental determinants of chronic pain are available[41], a few illustrative examples will be offered here. Regarding the health care system, pain behaviors are frequently reinforced by multiple visits to physicians and emergency room settings, the prescription of pain-relieving medications on a complaint-contingent basis, and the use of a work-to-tolerance model in rehabilitation and physical therapy activities. Alternative approaches generated by the behavioral intervention model include contracting by patients and physicians for specified, time-limited contact to discuss and reinforce achievement of treatment goals rather than symptoms and complaints[125], gradually withdrawing abused analgesic medications and administering them on a time-contingent basis, and using rest as a reward to reinforce attaining performance quotas in rehabilitational activities such as walking and exercises.

Attention to pain behaviors and complaints from spouse and family members frequently reinforces and maintains these behaviors. An often helpful psychological intervention is behaviorally based marital counseling[125] in which the spouse is instructed to ignore bids for help or complaints of pain and to provide high levels of attention and praise for coping and acceptable behaviors. The patient is told not to expect care from the spouse during pain episodes, but is encouraged to employ self-management strategies to control pain and discomfort.

The third category of environmental determinants of chronic pain includes avoidance behaviors and behavioral deficits such as excessive downtime (nonproductive time spent sitting or lying down), withdrawal from vocational, avocational, and social activities, and associated use of unnecessary appliances and prosthetic devices such as braces, canes, splints, or neck collars. Here the psychologist can be a useful behavioral consultant to other clinical specialists such as orthopedists, physiatrists, physical and occupational therapists, and vocational counselors. For example, effective behavioral strategies include assisting in setting and recording goals for activity, exercise, and social interaction, as well as establishing a time-contingent withdrawal schedule for unnecessary prosthetic devices. Likewise, the psychologist may suggest a gradual return to the work setting and assist the patient in constructing a work schedule that intersperses periods of work and activity with periods of rest. These interventions require close collaboration across the several disciplines involved in managing the pain patient and contribute to increased integration and communication among members of the treatment team.

The combination of medical management approaches and behaviorally oriented psychological methods has produced an effective and economical means of treating the complex problem of chronic pain. Although the evaluative and therapeutic approaches discussed in this chapter have proven useful to a majority of patients, a number of issues deserve the attention of clinicians and researchers interested in this field. One relates to the group of patients not significantly helped by established pain clinics, a segment reported by different centers to vary from 14 percent to 56 percent on follow-up.[10] Only a few studies address this group of dissatisfied or problem patients[126–128], and little is known about their psychological or behavioral features. Furthermore, there are no reports of treatment programs systematically trying to identify or remediate problem patients and determining subsequent effects on therapeutic outcome. A related issue is that of identifying which individuals in the population of acute pain patients progress to chronic pain status. This has a particular economic import for industry and insurance carriers. The combination of identifying behavioral or psychometric markers for patients at risk of developing a chronic pain syndrome and early intervention programs for such individuals would be very valuable. Developing educational and stress management programs for specific populations at risk for back injury, such as hospital employees[129], represents an important start in this direction.

A second area of future development relates to the increasing understanding of psychological and behavioral heterogeneity among the chronic pain population[130] and the need to devise treatment strategies that match psychological styles and needs. Although some attention has been paid to this issue in other areas such as anxiety reduction or smoking cessation[131, 132], most treatment programs for chronic pain appear to impose prepackaged interventions on all participants. Controlled outcome research into the interaction of psychological factors (e.g., cognitive-style variables such as locus of control or field-dependence-independence) and mode of treatment intervention (e.g., biofeedback versus transcutaneous electrical stimulation) would be useful in developing effective treatment packages.

Finally, of current and future interest is the development of evaluation and treatment programs for specific patient populations with chronic pain. Psychological and behavioral methods initially employed primarily with low back pain patients have been extended to those with facial pain[125,133], cancer pain[37,134], headache[135], and rheumatoid arthritis.[136] Continued controlled research to identify optimal intervention packages for these subgroups of chronic pain patients is clearly needed.

REHABILITATION

Ideally, the ultimate goal of pain management would be the patient's total and complete rehabilitation to premorbid lifestyle. This would include physical activity restoration and social reintegration up to and including the return to productive employment. In the long run it is likely that patients can be restored to a suitable physical condition and, with the appropriate coping/adaptive skills, can accommodate to their pain. Unfortunately, some of these patients who responded so favorably to treatment may encounter difficulties in achieving complete rehabilitation because of conflicts that arise from the encroachment of the litigation and/or compensation system on their lives. The fact that such patients may not be successfully rehabilitated for these last-mentioned reasons supports the concept that the treatment program *must* encompass not only treatment for the causes of the patients' physical pain, but also consider all of the complications that have ensued in their life related to that pain.

It can only be hoped that in the future more realistic, beneficial social programs for financial support, reeducation, retraining, lifestyle reorientation, work hardening, and return to the work site can be forthcoming.[137] By implication, the multidisciplinary approach to chronic pain should include social workers, public health nurses, among others, as these specialists will be the most adept at guiding the rehabilitating patient through the maze of social reentry programs, thereby maximizing the likelihood of successful treatment. It is not unexpected that pain center personnel will be increasingly prevailed upon by members of the legal profession for consultation and expert witness testimony. Pain must be consistently presented as the extremely complex phenomenon that it is, and the difficulties of its evaluation and management clearly stated.

CONCLUSION

Pain is clearly an intriguing and complex phenomenon that transcends the traditional physical realm of sensation. Although the management of acute pain is almost routinely effective, the evaluation and subsequent management of patients with chronic, ongoing pain is less successful. Referring physicians and consultants must demonstrate an all-encompassing attitude in approaching such patients. The pitfalls of the usual evaluation of chronic pain must be avoided and the philosophy that the patient is primarily responsible for carrying out the treatment program manifest. After a systematic and thorough evaluation of the patient's history, physical examination findings, and available laboratory studies, one must make a consummate diagnosis as to the etiologies of the patient's pain. Once this has been achieved and explained to the patient, the rationale for the creative treatment program must be discussed and the therapy implemented. Just as the patient must have an understanding of the suspected cause of pain and factors contributing to its perpetuation, so is the patient entitled to an honest, compassionate discussion of the rationale for the treatment options chosen.

Basically the pain can be expected to be decreased through the use of some combination of medications, surgery, nerve block techniques, and stimulation modalities. As the pain is diminished, the patient can be introduced to physical rehabilitation programs that aim to reverse the detrimental consequences of prolonged inactivity and restrictions induced by pain. It is likely that a decrease in pain and an increased capability to perform at least the activities of daily living will markedly improve the patient's attitude and outlook. However, there are those patients in whom the reality of residual chronic pain is not well tolerated. It is these patients who will require, at a minimum, periodic physician input for emotional support and encouragement. A smaller percentage of patients will require formal psychotherapeutic intervention to maximize their abilities to control pain and to cope with its persistent existence. The ultimate rehabilitation of the patient will be influenced by many medical, physical, iatrogenic, psychosocial, economic, and personal factors.

It behooves all specialists in clinical health care to understand the dimensions of pain, the depth to which it can penetrate the patient's existence, and the fundamental aspects of pain evaluation and management. Thereby, it is hoped that the devastation of the patient and the subsequent impact of "pain" on society and health care resources can be lessened. This chapter aims to help health care professionals establish a proper perspective for pain, gain insight into contemporary evaluation concepts, become enlightened about modern treatment concerns, and be confident that no one has all of the answers for every patient's pain problems. Even the multidisciplinary model, which attempts to leave no stone unturned, does not guarantee successful management, when success is rigidly defined as complete relief of pain and total restoration of lifestyle. When the less lofty but significant goals of decreased pain and increased function are accepted as success, many more patients and health care professionals will find satisfaction in the management of chronic pain.

REFERENCES

1. Melzack R, Wall PD: Pain mechanisms: a new theory. Science 150:971:–979, 1965.
2. Bonica JJ: Introduction, Evaluation and Treatment of Chronic Pain. Edited by Aronoff GM. Baltimore-Munich: Urban & Schwarzenberg, 1985, pp xxxi–xiiv.
3. Bonica JJ: History of pain concepts and pain therapy. Sem Anesth 4(3):189–208, 1985.
4. Mersky H: Classification of chronic pain. Descriptions of chronic pain syndromes and definition of pain terms. Pain DB (Suppl. 3): S1–S225, 1986.
5. Rowlingson JC: Pain syndromes: diagnosis and treatment. 1984 Annual Refresher Course Lectures, American Society of Anesthesiologists, Inc., Chicago, 1984, p110(i–vii).
6. Bonica JJ: Introduction (to narcotic analgesics in the treatment of cancer and postoperative pain). Acta Anaesth Scand (Suppl 74) 26:5–10, 1982.
7. Reuler JB, Girard DE, Nardone DA: The chronic pain syndrome: misconceptions and management. Ann Intern Med 93:588–596, 1980.
8. Levine J: Pain and analgesia: The outlook for more rational treatment. Ann Intern Med 100:269 –276, 1984.
9. Ng LKY: New approaches to the treatment of chronic pain: A review of multidisciplinary pain

clinics and pain centers. NIDA Research Monograph 36, NIDA, Washington, D.C., 1981.
10. Spielman FJ, Ghia JN: Pain control teaching in anesthesia residencies. Reg Anesth 8:154–157, 1983.
11. Melzack R: Recent concepts of pain. J Med 13:147–160, 1982.
12. Melzack R, Wall PD: The Challenge of Pain. New York: Basic Books, 1982.
13. Loeser JD: Pain due to nerve injury. Spine 10:232–235, 1985.
14. Kruger L, Mantyh PW: Changing concepts in the anatomy of pain. Sem Anesth 4(3):209–217, 1985.
15. Liebeskind JC, Sherman JE, Cannon JT, Terman GW: Neural and neurochemical mechanisms of pain inhibition. Sem Anesth 4(3):218–222, 1985.
16. Abram SE: Pain pathways and mechanisms. Sem Anesth 4(4):267–274, 1985.
17. Nayman J: Measurement and control of postoperative pain. Ann Roy Coll Surg Engl 61:419–426, 1979.
18. Twycross RG: The relief of pain in far-advanced cancer. Reg Anesth 5(3):2–11, 1980.
19. Marks RM, Sachar EJ: Undertreatment of medical inpatients with narcotic analgesics. Ann Intern Med 78:173–181, 1973.
20. Porter J, Jick H: Addiction is rare in patients treated with narcotics. N Engl J Med 302:123, 1980.
21. Angell M: The quality of mercy. N Engl J Med 306:98–99, 1982.
22. Giddon DB, Rabinovitz SL: The psychological aspects of treatment of chronic pain patients. Reg Anesth 5(3):16–23, 1980.
23. Carron H: Pain Assessment and Narrative, Charlottesville: University of Virginia, 1983.
24. Pawlicki RE, Bettinger R, Colvin DF, Henrick W, Knapp RB: Use of a comprehensive pain questionnaire to answer the question "who are chronic pain patients?" Paper presented at the American Pain Society, San Diego, California, 1979.
25. Lundeen TF, Turner SP, Toomey TC: Design and implementation of a microcomputer database management system for a pain clinic. Paper presented at 4th World Congress on Pain of the IASP, Seattle, Washington, 1984.
26. Scott J, Huskisson EC: Graphic representation of pain. Pain 2:175–184, 1976.
27. Melzack R: The McGill Pain Questionnaire: Major properties and scoring methods. Pain 1:277–299, 1975.
28. Ransford AO, Cairns D, Mooney V: The pain drawing as an aid to the psychologic evaluation of patients with low back pain. Spine 1:127–134, 1976.
29. Derogatis L: The SCL-90, Baltimore, Maryland, 1975.
30. Zung WWK: A self-rating depression scale. Arch Gen Psychiatry 12:63–70,1965.
31. Taylor IA: A personality scale of manifest anxiety. J Abnormal Soc Psychol 48:285–290, 1953.
32. Holmes TH, Rahe RH: The social readjustment rating scale. J Psychosom Res 2:213–218, 1967.
33. Levitt SR: The chronic pain battery, Pain Resource Center, Durham, North Carolina, 1983.
34. Pilowsky I, Spence ND: Patterns of illness behavior in patients with intractable pain. J Psychosom Res 19:279–287, 1975.
35. Carron H: Headache Questionnaire. Charlottesville: University of Virginia, 1981.
36. Lundeen, TF: The TMJ Scale. Pain Resource Center, Durham, North Carolina, 1983.
37. Bradley JJ: Severe localized pain associated with the depressive syndrome, Br J Psychiat 109:741–745, 1963.
38. Haber JD, Roos C: Traumatic events in chronic pain patients. PRN Forum Pain Research News 4:1–2, 1985.
39. Fordyce WE, Brena SF, Holcomb RJ, DeLateur BJ, Loeser JD: Relationship of patient semantic pain descriptions to physician diagnostic judgments, activity level measures, and MMPI. Pain 5: 293–303, 1978.
40. Klein RM, Charlton JE: Behavioral observation and analysis of pain behavior in critically burned patients. Pain 9:27–40, 1980.
41. Fordyce WE: Behavioral Methods for Chronic Pain and Illness. St. Louis: Mosby Press, 1976.
42. Keefe FJ, Wilkins RH, Cook WA: Direct observation of pain behavior in low back pain patients during physical exam. Pain 20:59–68, 1984.
43. Swanson DW, Maruta T, Swenson WM: Results of behavior modification in the treatment of chronic pain. Psychosom Med 41:55–61, 1979.
44. Rybstein-Blinchick E: Effects of different cognitive strategies in the chronic pain experience. J Behav Med 2:93–102, 1979.
45. Block AR: An investigation of the response of the spouse to chronic pain behavior. Psychosom

Med 43:415–422, 1981.
46. Sanders SH: Toward a practical instrument system for the automatic measurement of "up-time" in chronic pain patients. Pain 9:103–109, 1980.
47. Sanders SH: Assessment of up-time in chronic low back pain patients: comparison between self-report and automated measurement systems. Paper presented at Association for Advancement of Behavior Therapy, New York, 1980.
48. Nouwen A, Bush C: The relationship between paraspinal EMG and chronic low back pain. Pain 20:109–123, 1984.
49. Collins GA, Cohen MJ, Maliboff BD, Schandler SL: Comparative analysis of paraspinal and frontalis EMG, heart rate and skin conductance in chronic low back pain patients and normals to various postures and stress. Scand J Rehab Med 14:39–46, 1982.
50. Cram JR, Steger JC: EMG scanning in the diagnosis of chronic pain. Biofeedback and Self-Regulation 8:229–241, 1983.
51. Hoyt WH, Hunt HH, DePouw MA, Bard D, Shaffer F, Passias JN, Robbins DH, Runyon DD, Semrad SE, Symonds JD, Watt KC: Electromyographic assessment of chronic low-back pain syndrome. J Am Osteopath Assoc 80:57–59, 1981.
52. Aronoff GM: The use of non-narcotic drugs and other alternatives for analgesia as a part of a comprehensive pain management program. J Med 13:191–202, 1982.
53. Rowlingson JC, Stehling L: Anesthesia update#10: the evaluation and treatment of the patient with chronic pain. Orthop Rev 11:79–85, 1982.
54. Amadio P Jr: Peripherally acting analgesics. Am J Med 77(3A):17–26, 1984.
55. Inturrisi CE: Role of opioid analgesics. Am J Med 77(3A):27–37, 1984.
56. Stimmel B: Pain, analgesia, and addiction: an approach to the pharmacologic management of pain. Clin J Pain 1:14–22, 1985.
57. Beaver WT: Combination analgesics. Am J Med 77(3A):38–53, 1984.
58. Ready LB, Sarkis E, Turner JA: Self-reported versus actual use of medications in chronic pain patients. Pain 12:285–294, 1982.
59. Turner JA, Calsyn DA, Fordyce WE, Ready LB: Drug utilization patterns in chronic pain patients. Pain 12:357–363, 1982.
60. McNairy SL, Maruta T, Ivnik RJ, Swanson DW, Ilstrup DM: Prescription medication dependence and neuropsychologic function. Pain 18:169–177, 1984.
61. Khantzian EJ, Mckenna GJ: Acute toxic and withdrawal reactions associated with drug use and abuse. Ann Intern Med 90:361–372, 1979.
62. Simon LS, Mills JA: Non-steroidal anti-infllammatory drugs. N Engl J Med 302:1179–1185, 1980.
63. Simon LS, Mills JA: Non-steroidal anti-inflammatory drugs. N Engl J Med 302:1237–1243, 1980.
64. Henrich WL: Nephrotoxicity of non-steroidal anti-inflammatory agents. Am J Kidney Dis 2:478–484, 1983.
65. Stillman MT, Napier J, Blackshear JL: Adverse effects of non-steroidal anti-inflammatory drugs on the kidney. Med Clin North Am 68:371–385, 1984.
66. Hollister LE: Medical intelligence-tricyclic antidepressants (part 1). N Engl J Med 299:1106–1109, 1978.
67. Hollister LE: Medical intelligence-tricyclic antidepressants (part 2). N Engl J Med 299:1168–1172, 1978.
68. Rosenblatt RM, Reich J, Dehring D: Tricyclic antidepressants in treatment of depression and chronic pain: analysis of the supporting evidence. Anesth Analg 63:1025–1032, 1984.
69. Ward NG, Bloom VL, Friedel RO: The effectiveness of tricyclic antidepressants in the treatment of co-existing pain and depression. Pain 7:331–342, 1979.
70. Keeri-Szanto M: The mode of action of promethazine in potentiating narcotic drugs. Br J Anaesth 33:422–431, 1961.
71. Nathan PW: Chlorprothixene (Taractan) in post-herpetic neuralgia and other severe chronic pains. Pain 5:367–372, 1978.
72. Kanner R: Psychotropic drugs in the management of pain. Curr Concepts Pain 1(2):11–15, 1983.
73. Foley KM: Adjuvant analgesic drugs in cancer pain management, In: Aronoff GM(ed) Evaluation and Treatment of Chronic Pain. Baltimore-Munich: Urban & Schwarzenberg, 1985, pp 425–434.

74. Beaver WT: Management of cancer pain with parenteral medication. JAMA 244:2653–2657, 1980.
75. Foley KM: The treatment of cancer pain. N Engl J Med 313:84–95, 1985.
76. Bennett RL, Batenhorst RL, Graves D, et al.: Patient-controlled analgesia: A new concept of postoperative pain relief. Ann Surg 195:700–705, 1982.
77. Graves DA, Foster TS, Batenhorst RL, et al.: Patient-controlled analgesia. Ann Intern Med 99: 360–366, 1983.
78. White PF: Patient-controlled analgesia: A new approach to the management of postoperative pain. Sem Anesth 4(3):255–266, 1985.
79. Hameroff SR, Carlson GL, Brown BR: Ilioinguinal pain syndrome. Pain 10:253–258, 1981.
80. Young RF: Surgical role in the relief of pain. Sem Anesth 4(4):323–331, 1985.
81. Freidberg SR: The neurosurgeon's approach to pain, In: Aronoff GM. (ed) Evaluation and Treatment of Chronic Pain. Baltimore-Munich: Urban & Schwarzenberg, 1985, pp319–331.
82. Coggeshall RE, Applebaum ML, et al.: Unmyelinated axons in human ventral roots: a possible explanation for the failure of dorsal rhizotomy to relieve pain. Brain 98:157–166, 1975.
83. Rowlingson JC, Chalkley JD: Common pain syndromes–diagnosis and management. Sem Anesth 4(3):233—230, 1985.
84. Ramamurthy S, Winnie AP: Regional anesthetic techniques for pain relief. Sem Anesth 4(3):237 –246, 1985.
85. Ghia JN, Toomey TC, Mao W, Duncan G, Gregg JM: Towards an understanding of chronic pain mechanisms: the use of psychological tests and a refined differential spinal block. Anesthesiology 50:20–25, 1979.
86. Rowlingson JC: Current concepts of postoperative pain. Infect Surg 3(7):527–535, 1984.
87. Pflug AE, Murphy AM, Butler SH, et al.: The effects of postoperative peridural analgesia on pulmonary therapy and pulmonary complications. Anesthesiology 41:8–17, 1974.
88. Noller DW, Gillenwater JY, Howards SS, Vaughan ED Jr: Intercostal nerve block with flank incision. J Urol 117:759–761, 1977.
89. Goulding FJ: Penile block for postoperative pain relief in penile surgery. J Urol 126:337, 1981.
90. Cousins MJ, Mather LE: Intrathecal and epidural administration of opioids. Anesthesiology 61: 276–310, 1984.
91. Findler G, Olshwang D, Hadani M: Continuous epidural morphine treatment of intractable pain in terminal cancer patients. Pain 14:311–315, 1982.
92. Coombs DW: New approaches to chronic pain therapy. Sem Anesth 4(4):287–299, 1985.
93. Benzon HT: Epidural steroid injections for low back pain and lumbosacral radiculopathy. Pain 24:277–295, 1986.
94. Berman AT, Garbarino JL Jr, Fisher SM, Bosacco SJ: The effects of epidural injection of local anesthetics and corticosteroids on patients with lumbosciatic pain. Clin Orthop Rel Res 188:144–151, 1984.
95. Boas RA: Sympathetic blocks in clinical practice, In: Stanton-Hicks M(ed) International Anesthesiology Clinics—Winter 1978. Boston: Little, Brown, 1978, pp 149–182.
96. Rowlingson JC: The sympathetic dystrophies, In: Warfield C, Stein J. (eds) International Anesthesiology clinics. Boston: Little, Brown, 1983, pp117–129
97. Wang JK, Erickson RP, Ilstrup DM: Repeated stellate ganglion blocks for upper-extremity reflex sympathetic dystrophy. Reg Anesth 10:125–128, 1985.
98. Wang JK, Johnson KA, Ilstrup DM: Sympathetic blocks for reflex sympathetic dystrophy. Pain 23:13–17, 1985.
99. Lund PC: The role of analgesic blocking in the management of cancer pain: current trends, a review article. J Med 13:161–182, 1982.
100. Brechner TF: The management of pain associated with malignancy. Sem Anesth 4(4):313–322, 1985.
101. Edwards WT, Habib F, Burney RG, Begin G: Intravenous lidocaine in the management of various chronic pain states: A review of 211 cases. Reg Anesth 10:1–6, 1985.
102. Long DM: Stimulation of the peripheral nervous system for pain control. Clin Neurosurg 31: 323–343, 1983.
103. Vincent CA, Richardson PH: The evaluation of therapeutic acupuncture: concepts and methods. Pain 24:1–13, 1986.
104. Richardson PH, Vincent CA: Acupuncture for the treatment of pain: a review of evaluative research. Pain 24:15–40, 1986.

105. Mannheimer JS, Lampe GN: Clinical Transcutaneous electrical Nerve Stimulation. Philadelphia: FA Davis, 1984.
106. Solomon RA, Viernstein MC, Long DM: Reduction of postoperative pain and narcotic use by transcutaneous electrical nerve stimulation. Surgery 87:142–146, 1980.
107. Tyler E, Caldwell C, Ghia JN: Transcutaneous electrical nerve stimulation: An alternative approach to the management of postoperative pain. Anesth Analg 61:449–456, 1982.
108. McGuire EJ, Shi-Chun Z, Horwinski ER, Lytton B: Treatment of motor and sensory detrusor instability by electrical stimulation. J Urol 129:78–79, 1965.
109. Mannheimer C, Carlsson CA, Emanuelsson H, et al.: The effects of transcutaneous electrical nerve stimulation in patients with severe angina pectoris. Circulation 71:308–316, 1985.
110. Pflug AE, Bonica JJ: Physiopathology and control of postoperative pain. Arch Surg 112:773–781, 1977.
111. Fordyce W, McMahon R, Rainwater G, et al.: Pain complaints–exercise performance relationship in chronic pain. Pain 10:311–321, 1981.
112. Linton SJ: The relationship between activity and chronic back pain. Pain 21:289–294, 1985.
113. Wilensky J: Physiatric approach to chronic pain, In: Aronoff GM(ed) Evaluation and Treatment of Chronic Pain. Baltimore-Munich: Urban & Schwarzenberg, 1985, pp 199–230.
114. Yeh C, Gonyea M, Lemke J, Volpe M: Physical therapy: evaluation and treatment of chronic pain, In: Aronoff GM (ed) Evaluation and Treatment of Chronic Pain. Baltimore-Munich: Urban & Schwarzenberg, 1985, pp 251–262.
115. Doke JJ, Crocker MF, Moletteire C, Doleys DM: Exercise quotas, anticipatory concern, and self-efficacy expectancies in chronic pain: A preliminary report. Pain 24:365–372, 1986.
116. Beecher HK: Anxiety and pain. JAMA 209:1080, 1969.
117. Egbert LD, Battit GE, Welch CE, Bartlett MK: Reduction of postoperative pain by encouragement and instruction of patients. N Engl J Med 270:825–827, 1964.
118. Flor H, Hage G, Turk DC, Koehler H: Efficacy of EMG biofeedback, pseudotherapy, and conventional medical treatment for chronic rheumatic low back pain. Pain 17:21–31, 1983.
119. Sovak N, Kunzel M, Sternbach RA, Dalessio DJ: Mechanisms of the biofeedback therapy of migraine: Volitional manipulation of the psychophysiological background. Headache 21:89–92, 1981.
120. Blanchard EB, Andrasik F, Applebaum KA, Evans DD, Myers P, Barron KD: Three studies of the psychologic changes in chronic headache patients associated with biofeedback and relaxation therapies. Psychosom Med 48:73–83, 1986.
121. Rice KM, Bianchard EB: Biofeedback in the treatment of anxiety disorders. Clin Psych Rev 2: 557–577, 1982.
122. Toomey TC, Sanders S: Group hypnotherapy as an active control strategy in chronic pain. Am J Clin Hyp 26:20–25, 1983.
123. Copp LA: The spectrum of suffering. Am J Nurs 74:491–495, 1974.
124. Meichenbaum D, Turk D: The cognitive-behavioral management of anxiety, anger, and pain, In: Davidson PO (ed) Behavioral Management of Anxiety, Depression, and pain. New York: Bruner-Mazel, 1976, pp 1–34.
125. Toomey TC, Gregg JM, Raft DD: Behavioral management of chronic dental pain in an outpatient setting. Paper presented at North Carolina Psychological Association, Wilmington, North Carolina, 1974.
126. Rosomoff HL, Green C, Silbret M, Stelle R: Pain and low back rehabilitation program at the University of Miami School of Medicine, In: Ng LKY (ed) New Approaches to Chronic Pain: A Review of Multidisciplinary Pain Clinics and Pain Centers. NIDA Research Monograph 36. Washington, D.C.: NIDA, 1981, pp 92–111.
127. Seres JL, Painter JR, Newman RI: Multidisciplinary treatment of chronic pain at the Northwest Pain Center, In: Ng LKY (ed) New Approaches to Chronic Pain: A Review of Multidisciplinary Pain Clinics and Pain Centers. NIDA Research Monograph 36. Washington, D.C.: NIDA, 1981, pp 41–65.
128. Swanson DW, Swenson WM, Maruta T, Floreen AC: The dissatisfied patient with chronic pain. Pain 4:367–378, 1978.
129. Schwartz DP, DeGood DE, Mohr EM, Bauerle JA, Rowlingson JC: Can back pain be prevented in hospital employees? Preliminary findings from a comprehensive prevention and rehabilitation program. Paper presented at the 4th World Congress on Pain of the IASP, Seattle, Washington, 1984.

130. Bradley LA, Prokop LK, Margolis R, Gentry WD: Multivariate analyses of the MMPI profiles of low back pain patients, J Behav Med 1:253–272, 1978.
131. Best J, Steffy R: Smoking modification procedures tailored to subject characteristics. Behav Ther 2:177–191, 1971.
132. Goldfried MR: Psychotherapy as coping skills training, In Mahoney MJ (ed) Psychotherapy Process: Current Issues and Future Directions. New York: Plenum, 1980.
133. Keefe FJ, Dolan E: Pain behavior and pain coping strategies in low back pain and myofascial pain dysfunction syndrome patients. Pain 24:49–56, 1986.
134. Hilgard JR, LeBaron S: Hypnotherapy of Pain in Children with Cancer. Los Altos: Kaufmann Press, 1984.
135. Mitchell KR, White RG: Behavioral self-management: an application to the problem of migraine headaches. Behav Ther 8:213–222, 1977.
136. McDaniel LK, Anderson KO, Bradley LA, Young RA, Turner CA, Agudelo CA, Keefe FJ: Development of an observation method for assessing pain behavior in rheumatoid arthritis patients. Pain 24:165–184, 1986.
137. Catchlove R, Cohen K: Effects of a directive return to work approach in the treatment of workman's compensation patients with chronic pain. Pain 14:181–191, 1982.

4. RESEARCH, EDUCATION, AND TRAINING

JOHN M. GREGG

The life blood of any health science discipline is an integrated program of research, education, and clinical training. The field of dolorology is no exception. However, it has only been in recent years that the study of pain and its pedagogic applications have been approached scientifically. For much of mankind's history, inquiry and teaching about pain was in the hands of the shaman and pain was often viewed by the ancients as punishment by the wrathful gods.[1] In medieval times the church was the locus of knowledge. Painful suffering was taught to be part of God's plan to prepare individuals for the after-life. In Renaissance times, Descartes proposed a mind-body separatism that unfortunately is still reflected in current attitudes about "real" physical and "imagined" psychological pain.[2] The important World War II observations of Beecher questioned the validity of mind-body dualism for the pain experience[3], and Melzack and Wall's monumental proposal in 1965 led to an explanation of the psychophysiologic continuity of pain.[4] Finally, with the introduction of the multidisciplinary pain clinic by Bonica, the stage was set for a research, teaching, and therapy environment in which the entire breadth of the pain experience as a disease process could be addressed in a scientific manner. With the formulation of the International Association for the Study of Pain, and the publication of specialized journals, *Pain* and *Clinical Pain*, dolorology was finally a discipline capable of scientific self-scrutiny.

Although it is generally agreed that the care of people with pain disorders is best done in an environment where there is scientific objectivity and the questioning critique by colleagues and students, more often this care is dictated by expediency, past practices, and financial pressures.

What, then, is the status of pain education and research? What has been the impact of the multidisciplinary center? What common problems persist? What are the logical models for future progress in education and research, and what is needed to achieve them?

PAIN RESEARCH

The past 25 years have witnessed near-explosive advances in pain research, both basic and applied-clinical, and in the worldwide dissemination of information. A review of pain-related publications from the *Index Medicus* in September 1961 yielded 42 listings. In September 1986 there were 962, more than a 1000 percent increase. In addition, a full library of books, brochures, tapes, and symposia publications is now available to the pain scientist-clinician. Two high-quality journals are now devoted to pain research[5,6], and pertinent articles are seen monthly in the specialty journals from virtually all clinical disciplines. Major scientific sessions on pain are found yearly in annual meetings such as the Neurosciences, American Association for the Advancement of Science, and the National Academy. In 1986 alone, more than 170 special symposia were advertised in the general medical and scientific literature. And the International Association for Study of Pain with its subsidiary national organizations such as the American Association for the Study of Pain sponsored over 35 symposia or major meetings in 1986.

Research training

Research training for the majority of scientists or clinicians interested in pain appears still to be carried out by traditional Ph.D. programs within the basic science disciplines such as neurophysiology, anatomy, pharmacology, neuroscience, psychology, and biomedical engineering.

Clinicians in specialty training programs, particularly anesthesiology, neurosurgery, neurology, family medicine, and psychiatry, have increasingly taken opportunities to be involved in ongoing pain research activities at many institutions. Unfortunately, the instances of formal rotations for such clinicians in established pain center research programs continue to be limited. Currently, 22 formal post-doctoral research fellowships are listed through the office of the International Association for the Study of Pain with opportunities for both basic and clinical research (See Appendix A at the end of this chapter).

Research funding

Research funding for pain-related research, although difficult to precisely define, has also expanded exponentially in the past 25 years. For example, the funds allocated by the National Institutes of Health (NIH) and National Science Foundation (NSF) for even peripherally related projects were on the order of less than $800,000. In 1986, NIH-funded pain research used intramural and extramural center programs, program project support, and individual grants that totaled in excess of

$15 million. Primary sources of funds for pain research have been the National Institutes of Health, especially the National Institute on Mental Health, the National Institute on Drug Abuse, National Institute on Dental Research, and the National Science Foundation (see Appendix B at the end of this chapter). Considerable support has also been obtained from private industry, particularly pharmaceutical companies. And increasingly, revenues from patient care have been diverted to ongoing research programs.

Research progress

Research progress in the past 25 years has relied on the premises that (1) because of the nature of the problem, pain research must reflect a continuum of basic to applied (clinical) research and (2) since dolorology is still a young and emerging science, its boundaries and personnel should not be restricted along traditional disciplinary lines. Both of these premises have been met in the environment of the pain center and to a lesser degree by the large program project format where scientists and clinicians from differing backgrounds are brought together for interchange, cross-fertilization, and innovation.

Current problems

There are many obstacles to continued progress in pain research. The funding base for the health sciences from traditional sources such as the federal government has not shown significant growth in the past decade. Pursuing research grants, especially by young clinicians with little research application backgound, is very competitive and sometimes intimidating. Grants are often restricted to supply and equipment categories and do not provide for the critical salaries of technicians and expert ancillary researchers who may be needed by a busy clinician. Unfortunately, current political trends appear to favor defense and geotechnological-oriented research rather than health. Competition for the research dollar and for demurred academic positions in institutions where long-term research might be carried out has become increasingly difficult, and morale among potential scientist-clinicians appears low at this time.

Certain recent trends in health care delivery also seem retrogressive in solving the more complex problems presented by chronic pain. Specifically, the proliferation of outpatient and ambulatory care clinics can bias the public and health care administrations toward the misconception that health problems worthy of funding have "quick fix" solutions. This approach is often incompatible with the more careful and thorough investigation and treatment required for chronic pain problems. The emergence of health maintenance organizations (HMOs) also mitigates to some degree against the needs of chronic pain management. Costs for effective programs in pain research and management can be expensive and are not easily predicted for a given patient. This is inconsistent with the requirements for cost predictions for both HMO and some Medicare-type programs.

Other problems relate to the ethics of pain research. Concerns about human experimentation remain an important issue in pain research, especially when they pertain to people with major pain problems who may not be able to make completely rational and informed decisions. Specific examples include children with pain disorders, mentally handicapped individuals, people experiencing pain who also have psychiatric illness, and individuals whose pain is so severe that they will submit to any form of potentially helpful therapy.[7–9]

Controversy also persists over the use of animals for any pain research.[10,11] The use of "higher intelligence" animals such as dogs, cats, and especially primates is questioned when used in pain-modeling studies.[12] Ironically, the most meaningful studies are those that approximate the human experience of pain suffering in the experimental animal, a concept that many people, scientists included, find unacceptable. Although alternatives such as computer modeling, use of "lower animals," and reliance on normal human volunteers all have merit, each may lack certain essentials of the pain experience that must be studied if scientific progress is to be made.[13]

Solutions

What then are the logical steps needed to assure continued progress in pain research? First, it would appear that a broader and more diverse financial base is needed, one that encompasses not only the traditional granting sources but also private industry, sponsorships by foundations, and revenues that are linked appropriately to patient care. An important key to these alternative sources may be public and industrial education about the potential for improved health care and cost effectiveness that could result from better understanding of pain and its therapies.

Opportunities for research should come from a spectrum of environments rather than a single resource. There is need for opportunities for young scientists in biological curricula at the secondary school level, the colleges, and of course professional schools such as medicine, dentistry, nursing, and osteopathy. In fostering research it should be realized that scientific progress in this field must come from diverse sources. Therefore, encouragement should be given to individuals in diverse disciplines and backgrounds, and access to pain research societies and scientific meetings must not become exclusive.

Because clinical research requires both patients and clinicians for its conduct, encouragement must be given to private as well as institutional clinicians to develop protocols, collect data, and present and publish findings. The model of the solitary clinician-scientist, although largely abandoned in favor of more complex and high-technology–dependent groups, has nevertheless historically been a source of important information and should be encouraged. Incentive programs for pain research should be encouraged from within the national associations of the various medical specialties. Most clinical organizations have research committees with discretionary funds for appropriate research. The most favorable and fruitful environment for the direction and nurture of pain research, however, would seem to be the multidisciplinary pain center(figure 4–1). The requirements for this environment would include (1) adequate patient population, (2) stable funding base, (3) administrative support and direction, (4) necessary clinical and

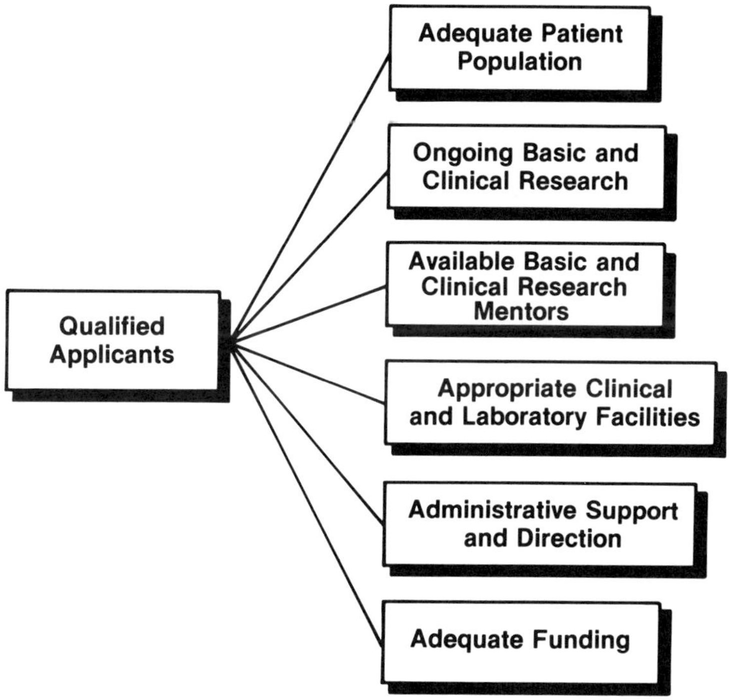

Figure 4–1. Components of the multidisciplinary pain research and education center

laboratory facilities and equipment, (5) availability of both clinical and basic research scientists, and (6) ongoing basic and clinical research projects.

Postdoctoral fellowships of this type have been sought mainly by medical or dental clinicians and by post-Ph.D. students, but other students could come from bachelor's degree programs such as nursing, physical therapy, and psychology. In addition, consideration could be given to educational recognition of advanced training such as the master's degree or to certification of the technical aspects of pain therapy.

PAIN EDUCATION AND TRAINING

In spite of the striking research breakthroughs in the understanding and management of pain in the past 25 years, actual awareness and application of these findings and principles by the general health care community lag far behind. Even at the most basic levels, such as the medical school curricula in the United States, the subject of chronic pain has not been given systematic attention. And at the critical level of advanced specialty training, recent surveys have shown that only 50 percent of trainees in residencies of anesthesiology are given direct experience with pain patients in a formal clinic setting.[14]

A concerted effort must be made to disseminate the significant findings and principles of pain science to four target groups: (1) health professionals, (2) basic scientists, (3) nonmedical health officials, and (4) the lay public.

Health professionals

Pain education must begin with a strong presence in the undergraduate schools of medicine, osteopathy, and dentistry. Basic concepts should reach allied professionals in nursing, physical, and occupational therapy, pharmacy, clinical psychology, social work, and medical technology. In addition, information must be carried to paramedical professionals in the clergy, sports medicine settings, nursing homes, hospice programs, and rehabilitation counseling. At another level, clinicians in medical specialty programs must be brought into contact with experienced dolorolgists and exposed to ongoing research in this field.

Clinical rotations, direct experience with pain patients, and an awareness of the now-extensive literature are essential. For established and private clinicians, there should be more opportunities for symposia and especially for "mini-residencies" in the multidisciplinary pain clinic setting.

Basic scientists

Basic scientists need to observe first-hand the clinical problems of pain to more effectively interface with clinicians in research. This process can take place at special symposia and at the group conference level of the multidisciplinary clinic, ideally at a weekly or monthly meeting when various consultants are directed toward clinical problems and controlled patient presentations are made. This process, of course, can also be integrated into less formal settings such as clinical rounds.

Health care officials

Nonprofessionals represent another important and untapped target population for pain education. Hospital directors, boards of trustees, insurance executives, politicians, and journalists, all are people in positions of authority to influence the support for research and pain health care itself. These workers should be made aware of the dimensions of the social and economic costs of chronic pain, estimated at over $55 billion in productivity lost yearly by full-time workers alone.[15]

General public

The general public must continue to be educated about advances made by pain scientists. The public should be informed of the relationship of pain to depression, drug abuse, the work force, family structure, and general principles of care. Inappropriate and ineffective therapies should also be discussed openly for public education. Curious citizens are best reached, of course, through television, although tapes, magazine, articles, and talks at Parent Teacher Associations, service organization meetings, and at community colleges all have potential for reaching the public. Ultimately, the support for research and better health care must come as a by-product of an informed public.

Finally, what should be the role of the dolorologist in the overall scheme of pain research, education, and patient care? It would seem logical that he or she would not be a substitute to whom all unsolved problems would be referred. The problems are simply too diverse, endemic, and complex. Rather, the pain specialist would best function as a director, consultant, and educator. He or she must therefore be a balance of scientist, clinician, teacher, and humanitarian to be effective.

In conclusion, tremendous strides have been made in the past 25 years in pain research and education. The multidisciplinary pain center has been an important but by no means the only driving force. Even though we have have seen research funding increase dramatically during this time, more recently the available support may be critically shrinking. The multidisciplinary pain center must continue in its role of leadership and reach out further to the broader medical community and lay public for new ideas, support, and cooperation.

REFERENCES

1. Procacci P: History of the pain concept. In: Kosterlitz HW, Terenivs LY (eds) Pain and Society. Dahlem Konferenzen, 1980, pp3–12.
2. Descartes R: L homme. Paris: Angot, 1644.
3. Beecher HK: Measurement of Subjective Responses. London: Oxford University Press, 1959.
4. Melzack R, Wall PD: Pain mechanisms: a new theory. Science 150:971, 1965.
5. Pain. Elsevier Science Publishers. P.O. Box 211 1000 AE, Amsterdam, The Netherlands.
6. The Clinical Journal of Pain. Raven Press Books Ltd. 1140 Avenue of the Americas, New York, NY 10036.
7. Bayer JE, Byers MC: Knowledge of pediatric pain: the state of the art. child Hlth Care 13:150–159, 1985.
8. Dworkin RH, Richlin DM, Handlin DS, Brand L: Predicting threshold response in depressed and nondepressed chronic pain patients. Pain 24:343–353, 1986.
9. Reading AE: Testing pain mechanisms in people in pain. In: Wall PD, Melzack R (eds). Textbook of Pain. Churchill-Livingstone, Edinburgh: 1984, pp 195–206.
10. Vyklicky L: Methods of testing pain mechanisms in animals. In: Wall PD, Melzack R (eds) Textbook of Pain. Churchill-Livingston, Edinburgh: 1984, pp 178–185.
11. Coderre TJ, Grimes RW, Melzack R: Deafferentation and chronic pain in animals: an evaluation of evidence suggesting autotomy is related to pain. Pain 26:61–84, 1986.
12. Cooper BY, Vierck CJ: Measurement of pain and morphine hypalgesia in monkeys. Pain 26:361–392, 1986.
13. Angier N: The electronic guinea pig. Discover 76–80, September 1983.
14. Spielman FJ, Ghia JN: Pain control teaching in anesthesia residencies.Reg Anesth 8:154–157, 1983.
15. Sternbach RA: Survey of pain in the United States: the nuprin report. Clin J Pain 2:49–53, 1986.

APPENDIX A: TRAINING OPPORTUNITIES IN PAIN RESEARCH AND TREATMENT

Reference: Louisa E. Jones, Executive Officer
International Association for the Study of Pain
909 NE 43rd Street, Room 306
Seattle, WA 98105, USA

Kasumi Arakawa, M.D., PH.D., Professor and Chairman
Department of Anesthesiology
University of Kansas Medical Center
39th and Rainbow Boulevard
Kansas City, KS 66103

Leonard Brand, M.D., Director, Pain Treatment Service
Columbia-Presbyterian Medical Center
622 West 168th Street
New York, NY 10032

Professor Michael J. Cousins
Department of Anesthesia and Intensive Care
Flinders Medical Centre,
Adelaide, South Australia 5042
Australia

Robert H. Dworkin, Ph.D., Pain Treatment Service
Columbia-Presbyterian Medical Center
622 West 168th Street
New York, NY 10032

W. Thomas Edwards, Ph.D, M.D.
University of Massachusetts Medical Center
Department of Anesthesiology
55 Lake Avenue, North
Worchester, MA 01605

Ronald J. Faust, M.D. Director, Educational Programs
Department of Anesthesiology
Mayo Clinic
200 First Street SW
Rochester, MN 55905

Theresa Ferrer-Brechner, M.D., UCLA Pain Management Center
Department of Anesthesiology
Los Angeles, CA 90024

J.N. Ghia, M.D., and J.D. Mann, M.D., Pain Clinic
The University of North Carolina, Departments of Anesthesiology and Neurology
Chapel Hill, North Carolina 27514

Ronald Kanner, M.D., Director Unified Pain Service
Montefiore Medical Center/ Albert Einstein College of Medicine
111 East 210th Street
Bronx, NY 10467

John D. Loeser, M.D.
University of Washington Pain Clinic RC-76
1959 N.E. Pacific Street
Seattle, WA 98195

Jim T. Long, M.D., Director of the Pain Clinic
Department of Anesthesiology
West Virginia Medical Center
Morgantown, WV 26505

APPENDIX B: PRIMARY SOURCES OF PAIN RESEARCH SUPPORT

National Institutes of Health; National Institute on Drug Abuse
5600 Fishers Lane
Rockville, MD 20857

National Institutes of Health; National Institute of Neurological and Communicative Disorders and Stroke
Federal Building, Room 714
Bethesda, MD 20892

National Institutes of Health
National Institute of General Medical Sciences;
Pharmacology Sciences Program
Westwood Building, Room 919
Bethesda, MD 20892

National Institutes of Health
National Institute of Dental Research
Craniofacial Anomalies, Pain Control and Behavioral Research
Westwood Building, Room 506
Bethesda, MD 20892

National Science Foundation
1800 G. Street NW
Washington, D.C. 20580

Professor Mirian Martelete, Pain Unit
Hospital de Clinicas de Porto Alegre
Rue Ramiro Barcelos, 2350
90000 Porto Alegre, Brazil

Donald B. Penzien, Ph.D., Dept. Psychiatry and Human Behavior
University of Mississippi Medical Center
2500 North State Street
Jackson, Mississsippi 39216

Professor P. Procacci, Servizio di Algologia, Cliinica Medica I
Viale Morgagni 85-50134
Firenze, Italia

Edward J. Resnick, M.D., Pain Control Center
Temple University Hospital
3401 North Broad Street
Philadelphia, PA 19140

John C.Rowlingson, M.D., Director Pain Management Center
Box 238, University of Virginia Medical Center
Charlottesville, VA 22908

Dr. Steven H. Sanders
Pain Control and Rehabilitation Institute of Georgia, Inc.
350 Winn Way
Decatur, GA 30030

Manjit K. Sihota, Director, Pain Control Center
University of Illinois at Chicago
1740 West Taylor Street
Chicago, Illinois 60680

Bruno Urban, M.D.
Box 3060, Duke University Medical Center
Durham, NC 27710

Russel P. Wall, M.D.
Georgetown University Pain Clinic
Georgetown University Hospital, Department of Anesthesiology
3800 Reservoir Rd.
Washington, D.C. 20017

Toshikatsu Yokota
Department of Physiology
Medical College of Shiga
Seta, Otsi 520-21
Japan

5. MANAGEMENT OF CHRONIC PAIN: WHAT HAVE WE ACHIEVED IN THE LAST 25 YEARS?

SRIDHAR V. VASUDEVAN

Pain continues to be one of the major symptoms for which individuals seek attention from the health care system. Although there is no uniformity regarding definition, theoretical explanations, management principles, or measurement of pain, the last 25 years have been characterized by increased interest in pain management and research.

The distinction between acute, biologically useful, time-limited pain and chronic pain, associated with no useful biological purpose and with significant physical, psychosocial alterations, has been recognized and accepted. Although several centers have reported successful results with multidisciplinary team management of patients with chronic pain, controversy exists regarding the best approach to such patients. Availability of pain clinics has increased, but accountability of successful outcome measures is in question. Measurement of program effectiveness continues to be a major issue in this day of cost-effective treatment and prospective payment.

In addition, several clinical questions remain unresolved. The issues of the relationship of depression and pain, litigation and pain, and the role of psychologic factors on pain and pharmacological manipulation of pain are still debated but are evolving and developing at a rapid rate. This chapter reviews the current literature and status in these selected areas.

ACUTE VERSUS CHRONIC PAIN

The recent literature reveals a preponderance of information and studies identifying the differences between acute pain and chronic pain. Acute pain is an unpleasant sensory, perceptual, emotional, and mental experience with associated autonomic, psychological, and behavioral responses provoked by acute disease or injury. It has been increasingly recognized that pain is a psychophysiological experience, involving not only nociception, the perception of noxious physical stimuli, but also the interpretation of these sensations as "painful" and evaluation of the pain as creating "suffering."[5,6,13,75] Engel, in 1959, emphasized that pain is the cardinal manifestation of illness and relief of pain is probably the most common demand by the patient upon the physician.[17] In spite of this importance of pain and the recognition of psychological and social factors in the pain phenomenon, the patient with persistent pain continues to baffle physicians in the health care system and to stress the knowledge of the physician and the economic resources of society.

Chronic and persistent pain imposes severe emotional, physical, economic, and sociological stresses on the patient, family, and society.[3,5,9,10,13] Unlike acute pain, individuals with chronic pain are often characterized by the presence of pain behaviors that cannot be explained by biomedical findings. Chapman emphasizes that to many individuals, pain becomes a lifelong companion and they attend to nothing else, pain becoming a force that disrupts the social, sexual, recreational, and vocational aspects of their lives.[10] Brena and Chapman emphasized the five *Ds* that are characteristic of individuals with chronic pain.[6] These are *dramatization* of complaints, *dysfunction* demonstrated by badges such as collars and braces, *drug* misuse, *dependency* on family and society, and *disability* that far exceeds the underlying biomedical findings.

Most chronic pain begins as an acute pain, often with an injury, inflammation, or surgical incision. Physicians continue to view chronic pain, in spite of acknowledged emotional problems, as acute pain and continue to approach it in this fashion. Bonica, who has contributed significantly to the recognition and understanding of chronic pain, defines chronic pain as that which persists beyond the usual course of an acute disease or reasonable time for an injury to heal or recurs at intervals for months or years.[5] Thus, chronic pain does not serve a usual biological function but imposes severe emotional, physical, economic, and social stresses on the patient and the family and is an expensive health care problem to society.[5,6,49,76]

Specialists in many fields, especially anesthesiology, neurosurgery, physiatry, orthopedics, and psychiatry, have shown increased interest in treating patients with the usual and prolonged complaints of pain. In addition to the difficulty of defining pain is the problem of arriving at the classification of pain syndromes. Crue provides a classification on underlying etiology and pathophysiology and classifies pain temporally.[13] Thus, he differentiates between *acute pain*, which lasts up to a few days in duration with the presumed nociceptive input; *subacute pain* of a few days to a few months in duration, non-emergency but treated like acute pain; *recurrent acute pain*, where there is recurrent or continued nociceptive input from underlying chronic pathological process; *ongoing acute pain* due to uncontrolled neoplastic disease with nociceptive input; *chronic benign nonneoplastic pain*, usually lasting more than six months with no known nocioceptive peripheral input but pain often made more severe by subsequent sensory input (and here is included "central pain") whereby patients seem to cope adequately; and, finally, *chronic intractable benign pain syndrome* (CIBPS), wherein chronic pain occurs with poor patient coping mechanisms and pain becomes the central focus of the patient's existence and there is no known nocioceptive peripheral input.[13] Pinsky defines the CIBPS as an ongoing problem with pain that (1) cannot be shown to be causally related to the here-and-now with any active pathophysiologic or pathoanatomic process; (2) has an antecedent history of generally ineffective medical and surgical intervention of the pain problem; and (3) has come to be accompanied by disturbed psychosocial functioning that includes the pain complaint and the epiphenomena that accompany it.[50] Black identified the chronic pain syndrome and provides a mnemonic SHAFT for the *s*ad, *h*ostile, *a*nxious, *f*rustrating patient, who *t*enaciously clings to the health care system.[4] Although pain is what the patient says it is, it should be recognized that pain is a personal and private sensation of hurt that may not be associated with a harmful stimulus. Several years ago Lewis described pain as "any experience, whether physical or mental, which the patient dislikes."

Chronic pain syndrome

The patient with chronic pain syndrome or CIBPS presents with persistent symptoms of pain, reveals significant dependence on analgesic medications, has become unresponsive to multiple surgical procedures, demonstrates no clear organic pathology, reveals sleep pattern alterations with disturbance of the circadian rhythm, and is unresponsive to the usual medical, surgical, and psychiatric management.[4, 5, 13, 49, 50] Other environmental, familial, and social factors affect pain.

The patient with chronic pain syndrome or chronic intractable benign pain syndrome has the following characteristics:[5, 50, 76]

1. Ongoing pain not related to neoplastic disease or to a significant pathophysiological mechanism to explain ongoing pain and suffering,
2. Treatment with most, if not all, applicable medical and surgical techniques, with no relief or only transient relief,
3. Chronic pain as a central focus of thoughts and behaviors, which disrupts and destroys the psychosocial existence,
4. Associated drug dependency involving opioids, hypnotics, or tranquilizers,
5. Withdrawal from social and functional activities and from the social role whether it be as homemaker, productive worker, parent, or spouse,

Chronic pain syndrome has multiple contributing factors including anxiety, depression, and environmental situations such as job loss or divorce. Chronic pain is without doubt the most disabling disease, causing not only a serious national health problem but also a serious economic problem.[5, 57] It is estimated that more than 60 million Americans are affected with chronic pain, at a cost to the U.S. economy of $40 to $50 billion annually, including medical services, lost work productivity, and compensation payments.[5] Frequently encountered in the patient with chronic pain is secondary gain, which includes economic and other factors such as attention-seeking or a way to terminate employment.

Chapman defines human pain as complex and includes three dimensions. The first is the noxious sensory input term *nociception*. The second dimension is the motivational emotional dimension wherein the person feels aroused, perhaps fearful, and eventually the conceptual or judgmental dimension wherein the patient integrates present experience with past experiences and specific expectations of the immediate situation.[5,57]

Reuler and co-workers point out that frequently the health care workers are forced to assign patients to either organic or psychogenic categories, which allows them to ignore the fact that behavior is governed or controlled by consequences and environment. They point to several observations in their analysis of the chronic pain syndrome and underscore the point that although it does not matter whether pain is "real," identifying the factors that influence pain is critical.[52]

Crue identifies the peripheralist and the centralist concept of chronic pain.[13] The *peripheralist* believes that chronic pain can be viewed basically as a continuation of the nociceptive input, as in the acute pain medical model, when for some reason the original cause of pain, which started the nociceptive input, continues "longer than expected," "longer than usual," or even "longer than seems reasonable." Thus, a peripheralist believes in continued peripheral input and that the patient therefore can be "eventually healed correctly and fixed right." The *centralist*, however, believes that with any tissue damage in acute pain, some type of central "memory of pain" is established that can be hypothetically conceptualized as a "reverberating circuit," "internucial pool," or "repetitive epileptiform firing" in the sensory networks of the central nervous system. Thus, under appropriate conditions, the patient's brain can generate and continue to signal pain even further upward to the "alarm bell" in the patient's "mind," which we refer to as a conscious awareness of self. The pain can become "chronic" after only a few days or several months.

This author's experience indicates the probable presence of both mechanisms, which may be acting together in any one case or continuing to exist in different proportions, in causing human suffering.

There continues to be association between stress and pain. In a recent study, Sternbach notes that greater stress and more "hassles" are associated with more frequent and more severe pains and that there is a positive relationship between stress and pain.[67]

Margolis recently surveyed internists and found that there was a high prevalence of chronic pain, with a majority of patients being female and over 55 years of age.[41] The survey also found that internists attended to the disorder with a restrictive range of treatments, that patient reactions often interfere with treatment, and that internists had little or no formal education in the treatment of this disorder.[41]

Chronic pain can be one of the most difficult and perplexing patient problems encountered by a physician. The disorder has disabling effects, not only on emotional well-being, social interactions, and vocational and marital relationships, but on the patient's entire psychological makeup.

Chronic pain is not only a problem for the individual patient but affects the family as well. Marital difficulties have been noted between chronic pain patients and their spouses in several studies. Moreover, the presence of psychiatric distress in the spouse may affect the symptoms managed in the patient with chronic pain. Shanfield and co-workers studied pain patients and their spouses and found a significant correlation between spousal psychological distress and high symptom levels in pain patients.[62] Because of this, it is recommended that spouses be evaluated routinely along with pain patients. Treatment of these symptoms made a major impact on the pain and associated behavior.

Chronic pain—A posttraumatic stress disorder?

Modlin has recently reviewed posttraumatic stress disorder (PTSD), emphasizing that it can occur after any major stress.[44] The essential feature of posttraumatic stress disorder is the development of characteristic symptoms after a psychologically traumatic event generally outside the range of everyday human experience. Symptoms include reexperiencing the traumatic event and numbing of responsiveness to, or reducing involvement with, the external world. In addition, a variety of autonomic, dysphoric, or cognitive symptoms can occur. Although PTSD is a specific syndrome, a variety of traumatic events and situations have been implicated as etiologic or precipitative. In a typical practice this may include a single unexpected accident on the highway, on the job, or at home.[44] Other stresses producing PTSD are natural catastrophes such as floods and earthquakes; calamaties such as fires, plane crashes, ship sinkings, and building collapses; military combat; and deliberately produced disasters such as prisoners of war barbarities, concentration camps, bombings, and torture. Frequently, symptoms include anxiety, phobic avoidance reaction, muscle tension, irritability, impaired concentration and memory, startle reaction, repetitive nightmares, sexual inhibition, and social withdrawal. A sudden frightening accident causing little or no physical damage is a more likely precipitant of this psychiatric disorder. Patients become vulnerable with frequent citations such as "I can't trust the world anymore." "I don't know when it will attack me."[44] Such similar reactions can be seen with chronic pain patients who become helpless and vulnerable. There are some similarities between PTSD and CIBPS, and between psychosomatic or psychophysiological reaction, including persistent low back pain, psychogenic pain, prolonged concussion syndrome, cardiac neurosis.[44]

Muse emphasizes the fact that chronic pain due to benign disease frequently has substantial psychosocial bases and responds well to treatment typically applied to stress-related disorders. He presents criteria for the diagnosis of a specific variety of chronic pain syndromes that have etiologic bases in posttraumatic stress.[47] In his study, he emphasizes that the prevalence of the posttraumatic chronic pain syndrome is substantial and that posttraumatic stress may play an important role in a significant fraction of the chronic pain patients seen in a pain clinic setting.[44, 47] However, he raises several questions:[47]

1. Are the pain and the syndrome generated primarily from peripheral changes such as muscular spasm with ischemia or is there psychogenic process involved?
2. Is every area of the body capable of having a stress-related posttraumatic chronic pain condition? The most common areas noted with such pain were low back and cervical regions as well as the limbs.
3. What is the frequency of the syndrome in the chronic pain population?
4. How significant is the effect of posttraumatic stress in explaining the long-term disabling nature of chronic pain? He emphasizes that some of the chronic pain is probably continued by, in addition to the stress-related component, operantly learned pain behavior, compensation neurosis, and so on.
5. What is the most effective treatment for this syndrome? If there is a component of the posttraumatic stress disorder, resolution of the stress disorder becomes an important part of chronic pain treatment along with the application of behavioral techniques, such as relaxation training, desensitization procedures, implosion approaches, and in vivo strategies.

Schottenfeld and Cullen discuss occupation-induced posttraumatic stress disorders and emphasize that approximately 20 percent of all patients referred to their clinic had persistent or recurrent somatic symptoms not explained on the basis of organic factors, psychologic impairment, or evidence of significant exposure to substances known to cause symptoms. Most patients had an atypical posttraumatic stress disorder, and many were characterized by attempts to avoid exposure to stressful situations, often limiting work, hobbies, and activities and revealing excessive concern about exposure.[59]

Chronic pain and depression

Depression is frequently associated with individuals with chronic pain. It is a characteristic feature of the patient with chronic pain syndrome and CIBPS.[16, 23, 32, 36, 63]

In a study of chronic pain and depression, Skevington found that pain sufferers report more depressive symptoms than controls, but there is no evidence to support the hypothesis that these symptoms are an expression of personal helplessness. Thus, higher levels of depressive symptoms in patients with chronic pain are not reflected by higher levels of self-blame or beliefs in the actions of others, so personal helplessness is discounted.[63]

There is disagreement about the nature of the relationship between chronic pain and depression. While some authors consider chronic pain masked depression, several authors have shown that chronic pain patients differ from patients with depression both in demographic characteristics and in their behavior patterns.[49,63] Depression can be a normal mood state, a symptom, or a syndrome. The distinction between feelings of sadness as a normal mood and abnormal depression is not always clear. In addition to disturbances of mood, the psychopathological disorder of depression involves a combination of neurovegetative symptoms (altered appetite, sleep, weight), cognitive symptoms (decreased self-esteem, guilt, hopelessness), psychomotor symptoms (agitation or retardation), and psychological changes (social withdrawal, indecisiveness, irritability).[36,55] Ranga Ramakrishnan and co-workers have shown that patients with depression, irrespective of the type, had more general somatic sensory symptoms than those patients without depression. Patients with major depression had more than those with minor or intermittent depression. There was no difference between patients with and without organic findings. Autonomic symptoms such as dry mouth, flushing, pallor, and tendency to sweat were seen in patients with major depression and least with those without depression.[36] These authors also showed that the anxious mood and other symptoms of anxiety are commonly seen in patients with chronic low back pain. The symptom of anxiety was more common in those with associated depression especially with major depression. The beneficial use of relaxation treatment and biofeedback in chronic low back pain patients may be due partially to the reduction in anxiety and in muscular tension.[23, 36]

Haley and co-workers report important sex differences in the relationships among depression, activity, and chronic pain. In female patients, depression was significantly related to self-reported pain severity. Depression did not correlate significantly with the activity patterns at nighttime for either men or women. Daytime reclining, an indication of inactivity, was frequently seen.[32] France and co-workers, studying the relationship between chronic pain and depression, noticed the incidence of major depression in the first-order relatives of those patients with depression to be higher than in those without depression. They raised the question about the notion of considering chronic pain simply as a variant of depression and suggest the possibility that the occurrence of major depression in chronic back pain might be related to general vulnerability to depression in these patients.[23] Thus, the etiological basis for the development of depression in chronic pain patients is still unclear. The authors conclude:[23]

1. Depression can be identified as a psychopathological disorder in the chronic pain patient.
2. Different subtypes of depression can further be identified in these patients.
3. Dexamethazone suppression test (DST) abnormalities are seen primarily in patients with major depression.
4. The familial incidence of major depression is higher in chronic pain patients with major depression than in chronic pain patients without major depression.
5. The phenomenology of depressive symptoms and symptoms of anxiety is different in these various subtypes of depression.

Dworkin and co-workers studied treatment responses in groups of chronic pain patients who were depressed and nondepressed.[16] In nondepressed patients, beneficial response to treatment was related to greater number of treatment visits, not receiving workers' compensation, fewer previous types of treatment, and low back pain. Patients with chronic pain and depression were more likely to benefit when they were employed at the beginning of the treatment and their pain was of a shorter duration. The reseachers conclude that activity and active involvement in the treatment are particularly important in the chronic patients who are depressed.[16]

The difference between depressed and nondepressed patients may be related to the cognitive disturbances frequently related to depression. Optimal prediction of treatment response in chronic pain may be achieved by dividing patients into groups based on psychological characteristics. The authors themselves point out that comparing depressed and nondepressed patients is too simplified an approach to chronic pain and depression.[16] This is because there may be several subgroups within this affective disorder of depression and several types of affective disorders are seen in patients with chronic pain.

MANAGEMENT OF CHRONIC PAIN

Reports from several pain management clinics/centers over the last three decades reveal a better understanding of the management of the individual with chronic pain. Many strategies are based on recognition of chronic pain as a psychobiologic phenomenon with social reinforcers. The treatment of acute pain, which has a biologic purpose and limited timeframe, has essentially used the principles of rest, appropriate analgesic medications, and provision of comfort and attention. The introduction of the group of nonsteroidal anti-inflammatory medications has added to the armamentarium of the physician and improved compliance. Narcotic medications on a "time-contingent" basis in appropriate and effective doses are recommended for the initial management of acute pain. Stimmel provides an excellent review of the pharmacological management of pain and provides guidelines for optimal use.[68]

The introduction of the gate control theory in 1965 and the discovery of endorphins in 1970 heralded new approaches in management of acute and chronic pain. The significant developments in this area are implantable electrodes to provide spinal cord stimulation (DCNS, dorsal column nerve stimulators) and deep brain stimulation (DBS). It is beyond the scope of this chapter to discuss these techniques in detail. The practical application of this knowledge of modulating pain perception is by the use of percutaneous or transcutaneous electrical nerve stimulation (TENS). The Gate Control Theory also provides a possible explanation for use and effectiveness of physical modalities such as heat and cold application and acupuncture.[6, 64]

Probably the most significant advance in chronic pain management is based on the recognition of psychologic and behavioral factors affecting the patient. The major principles in management of the chronic pain patient are now summarized:[4, 6, 8]

1. Cessation of narcotic intake and drug dependence or, at the least, changing from those known to be addictive.
2. Utilization of modalities: These include the use of nerve blocks to interrupt the nocioceptive pathways, electrical stimulation through transcutaneous methods, biofeedback for relaxation exercises, intra-articular injections of anesthetics and steroids, and sympathetic nerve blocks.
3. Encouraging activity: implemented by graded exercises and measured by "uptime versus downtime" with those recorded activities utilized for behavior modification. Exercises are utilized actively and passively to improve flexibility, strength, and endurance.
4. Psychological and cognitive-behavioral intervention with group therapy playing a predominant role. Operant conditioning principles using learning therapy play a significant part in most treatment approaches.
5. Minimizing vocalization of pain language; in a sense changing the "illness role" to a "well or health role."

Black[4], discussing the treatment of chronic pain syndrome, reports that narcotic medication is eliminated as higher thought processes are affected and that chronic users of analgesic medications report less pain after these medications are discontinued. Medications are eliminated using either a "pain cocktail" approach or a gradual reduction. Medication reduction is accomplished by changing from the "prn" approach to a "time-contingent" approach. Behavioral changes and pain-related environment manipulation use the learning principles of pain behavior modification and operant conditioning. Patients are also placed on a weight-reduction program and graded activity program; myofascial pain is treated with trigger points; nerve blocks may be used in an early case of chronic pain; and transcutaneous nerve stimulation may be used.

Margolis and co-workers[41], in their survey of treatment procedures used by internists with chronic pain patients, noted that supportive talk and non-psychoactive medications were most frequently used. In addition, exercise regimens, physical therapy, and psychoactive drugs were occasionally prescribed. The interventions least utilized were acupuncture and hypnosis. Biofeedback, surgery, nerve block, transcutaneous electrical nerve stimulation, and psychotherapy were also rarely employed as treatment modalities. The major problem in chronic pain treatment cited by the internists dealt with patient reactions: continued patient complaints, demands for faster results, refusal to accept the diagnosis of chronic pain, refusal of referral to a mental health professional, reluctance to consider nonsomatic causes, and demand for total relief.[41] The survey also noted little formal exposure during their medical training to the condition of chronic pain. The survey concluded that increasing the range of methods to treat chronic pain and dealing with the physician's personal reaction to the patient would improve the overall treatment for the chronic pain patient by the primary care physician.[41]

Chronic pain syndrome, although considered benign, is a serious psychosocial problem accompanied by a high prevalence of iatrogenic complications, including adverse drug reactions, ineffective surgical procedures, and excessive use of the health care resources. The modalities available for the physician in managing such patients include nonnarcotics and analgesics, psychoactive drugs, electrical stimulation, biofeedback relaxation techniques, hypnosis, behavior management, acupuncture, neurosurgical ablation, and a variety of injections and nerve blocks.[52]

Pinsky emphasizes that CIBPS, as defined by him, is a functionally true biosocial disorder and results from a psychosocial maladaptive human attempt to deal with life's stressors.[50] A good patient-therapist relationship, release of tension, cognitive learning, operant conditioning, suggestion, and persuasion are needed. Such counseling should emphasize to the patient that the pain problems are taken seriously and that the treatment program is designed for patients to assume the previous life roles without the use of medications but with a graded physical activity and incorporating several principles of nonpharmacological methods of pain management.

Vasudevan and Lynch review the dilemma faced by both the patient and physician in treating the patient with chronic pain that is not "curable."[75] They emphasize the need for physician ease in the counseling process and note that therapeutic benefits occur best with the active participation of the patient and family in setting and accomplishing reasonable goals. They provide guidelines for effective communication with the patient and family with chronic pain.[75]

We will now briefly review the major advances in therapeutic approaches to the patient with chronic pain. The reader is referred to other chapters in this book and the references[4, 6, 13, 49] for more detailed reading.

Nerve blocks

Neural blockade has been a mainstay in the management of pain. Techniques may be classified as subarachnoid, epidural, paravertebral somatic, sympathetic, peripheral, and local. While the actual chemical interruption of nerve conduction, as demonstrated by duration of sensory loss, lasts at most 18 to 24 hours, the subjective decrease in pain intensity reported by the patient lasts days, weeks, or even longer. This is explained on the "vicious circle of pain." According to this theory, noxious stimulation may trigger a series of segmental muscular and vasomotor responses, leading to regional "muscle spasms," ischemia, and edema, with a corresponding increase in regional noxious stimulation. By providing release of muscle contraction and increased blood flow to the painful area, nerve blocking breaks the vicious cycle and achieves prolonged relief. Brena, in a recent symposium, reviews the role of nerve blocks and chronic pain states with a review of clinical indications.[7]

In addition to the rationale based on the peripheralist viewpoint, where nocioceptive input is diminished or eliminated, nerve blocks may also function as a modality of hyperstimulation analgesia.[7] Thus, hyperstimulation may be viewed as "jamming" of patterned central neuronal activities. Brena, reviewing the role of conditioning and the responses to nerve blocking, notes poor relationship between such responses and the degree of objective medical findings.[7,10] Epidural blocks, cranial nerve blocks, sympathetic nerve blocks, and trigger point injections are frequently used in patients with chronic pain and have been shown, when used with behavioral approaches, to be effective in pain management.[3,7]

The positive effects of nerve blocking include:[7]

1. Nerve blocks alter sensory inputs and provide changes in painful perceptions.
2. Through repeated and periodic needling, deep tissue stimulation may achieve prolonged analgesia by altering central neuronal behaviors.
3. Changes in peripheral blood flow through sympathetic blockade may decrease the tissue edema and reestablish tissue homeostasis.
4. Nerve blocking may facilitate the patient's willingness to undertake a psychophysiological rehabilitation rather than a pure focus on emotional impairment.
5. Nerve blocking in a structured behavior modification program may enhance the patient-physician relationship and strengthen the physician role as an educator.

Brena also points out the negative effects of nerve blocking, including:[7]

1. If not properly used, nerve blocking could reinforce patients' convictions of illness and thus foster dependency and passivity.
2. Nerve blocks are an invasive technique with known complications and higher morbidity risks.

In a study of learned helplessness in response to nerve block in patients with chronic low back pain, Chapman and Brena report that patients with a fixed focus on their pain, high in pain-related behaviors and low in responsibilities, seem less likely to respond favorably to nerve blocks.[10]

In a recent article, Benzon reviews the role of epidural steroid injections.[3] Epidural steroid injections are one of the most effective nonoperative managements for back pain and are especially recommended in patients with signs and symptoms of nerve root irritation. Relief of pain is attributed to the anti-inflammatory effects of the steroid, and the depression of the hypothalmic-pituitary-adrenal axis by such epidural blocks lasts three weeks.[2] The mechanisms that explain prolonged benefit from local anesthetic injection include interruption of the sustained neural activity that produced and perpetuated the pain, relaxation of the paraspinal muscle spasm, and resolution of the probable reflex sympathetic dystrophy. In addition, local anesthetic epidural blockade interrupts the nerve supply to the facet joint capsule, thus permitting reduction of minor subluxation and relaxation of the muscles overlying the facet joint and allowing the dislocated articulated surface to move back into proper alignment. Thus, even mechanical causes of low back pain, especially those accompanied by signs of nerve root irritation, respond to epidural steroid injections. When compared to bedrest, epidural local anesthetic injection results in better improvement and shorten recovery.[3]

Transcutaneous nerve stimulation—Acupuncture

Transcutaneous electrical nerve stimulation (TENS) has been demonstrated to be effective in relieving pain in some chronic pain patients. Treatment success has ranged significantly but overall seems to be in the 40 percent range.[56] It is an effective addition to the treatment regimen but is not a substitute for the management of the drug abuse, pain behavior problems, or vocational and family problems common among chronic pain patients. Soric and Devlin review the use of transcutaneous nerve stimulation and provide some practical aspects and application.[64] The physiological principles of TENS include the gate control theory, central-biasing mechanism, release of endogenous morphines, and neural transmitters and peripheral blocking mechanisms.[67]

Richardson and Vincent review the role of acupuncture in the treatment of pain. Their review of the literature indicates good evidence from control studies for the short-term effectiveness of acupuncture in relieving clinical pain, with the reported therapeutic effect varying from 50 percent to 80 percent. In long-term follow-up data of six months or more, however, a substantial portion (usually half) of those initially helped suffer some degree of relapse.[54] The use of acupuncture in chronic pain remains unproven, and more and better studies are therefore needed before firm conclusions can be drawn.[54]

Psychological strategies

Fordyce pioneered the concept of chronic pain as a learned behavior and has outlined behavioral methods of management.[20,21] Many pain management programs utilize to some extent the principles of behavior modification.[6,20,76] Pain management programs, however, have begun to use a variety of psychological strategies, usually in combination. These include cognitive, behavioral, cognitive-behavioral, cojoint marital, family, group, psychoanalytic supportive psychotherapy, relaxation training, biofeedback, hypnosis.[19,49,71]

Fordyce reviews the concept of chronic pain and analyzes it from a learning point of view leading to a treatment program based on learning principles.[20] Treatment is designed to reduce medication and interference in activity because of pain and to increase performance in exercises, walking, and general activity level. Fordyce, Roberts, and Sternbach provide a response to the criticisms of behavioral treatment programs for chronic pain.[21] A criticism about behavioral management programs has been that the multifaceted pain programs have been unable to isolate the systematic relationships between program components and outcome variables. Fordyce, Roberts, and Sternbach thus emphasize that outcome studies have clearly shown their effectiveness, although not always with control groups. Fordyce also emphasizes that a *negative correlation* was found between exercise and pain complaints in chronic pain patients: The more they did the fewer the pain behaviors.[20,21] Thus pain behaviors may be little, if at all, related to inferences about underlying noxious stimulation. Thus, it is important to conceptualize behavioral treatment as treatment for *excess disability* instead of treatment of pain. Most patients with chronic pain indeed have excess disability—that is, they are more functionally disabled than one would expect.

Pain is not a disease; it is a symptom. Neither is chronic pain a disease; it is a syndrome. But over the years it has assumed the status of a pseudo-disease because it appears to have a "natural history" different from acute pain of similar location and intensity. Fordyce and co-workers emphasize that the behavioral approach assumes that pain behaviors may occur for a variety of reasons. The principle reasons are nociception, the adverse effects of disuse, and over guarding of involved body parts and contingent reinforcement from the environment.[20,21]

Gamsa and co-workers report the use of structured group therapy sessions in the treatment of chronic pain.[24] This group therapy method was moderately directed, integrating psychodynamic, cognitive, and behavioral models of therapy. Based on the experiences, they suggest the following:[24]

1. Closed-group formats may be more productive than open-ended formats, wherein new patients enter almost every week,
2. Physiotherapy and psychotherapy should be integrated into group sessions, thus using relaxation exercises as part of group therapy,
3. Videotape feedback should be used to provide objective evidence regarding the patient's interpersonal and illness behaviors.

Tan reviews the cognitive and the cognitive-behavioral methods for pain control. He reviews the frequently used psychological approaches to pain control, which include relaxation techniques, operant or external contingency management, hypnosis, modeling, biofeedback, provision of preparatory information, a variety of cognitive coping skills or strategies combined cognitive-behavioral interventions, Cognitive methods are those that directly attempt to modify thought process in order to attenuate pain. The underlying assumption of these approaches is that individuals' "cognitions" are appraisals of their environment and are therefore crucial determinants of their experience and emotions. In other words, our experiences and ideas can influence what we see or feel. Hence, faulty cognitions lead to negative experiences, including exacerbation of anxiety, depression, and pain. By altering such cognitions to more adaptive ones, negative experiences may be attenuated.[71]

Cognitive methods for pain control include the following strategies: providing information about an upcoming event involving potential discomfort, teaching patients to identify maladaptive responses to stress eliciting situations, and teaching patients to use specific cognitive coping skills like distraction, imagery techniques, and calming self statements.

Cognitive-behavioral methods are most comprehensive strategies and include not only cognitive interventions but also some behavioral components. These include relaxation, biofeedback, desensitization, external contingency management, modeling, and assertion training. Tan points out that the distinction made between cognitive and behavioral methods or cognitive-behavioral methods is arbitrary.[71] In his review, Tan notices methodological problems and the need for an outcome measure more dependent than pain per se and for more long term follow up studies.

The principal assumption of the cognitive theory is that psychological procedures, whatever their form, affect behavioral change by serving as means of creating and strengthening expectations of personal mastery or self-efficacy. An efficacy expectation refers to the conviction that one can successfully execute the behavior required to produce certain outcomes.[71]

Linton recently reviewed the relationship between activity and chronic back pain.[39] Activities were presumed to cause an increase in pain. If true, then chronic sufferers should regulate these activities and avoid participation when they have pain. A study showed that patients do not report a connection between activity and pain on global interview questions. There is no significant correlation between pain intensity and actual activity levels as measured by self-monitoring or observed behavior in test situations. This finding underscores the importance of a comprehensive behavioral assessment, as there was no direct correlation between activity levels and chronic pain intensity. This supports the operant view of chronic pain, namely, that environmental contingencies have an influence, so that verbal reports do not necessarily correspond with actual behavior. Chronic pain is a set of behaviors, all equally valid and important. What people say is just as important as what they do, even if the two do not always correspond.[20,39]

Fernandez reviews the cognitive coping strategies for pain and provides a classification system. He divides the strategies into three broad categories—imagery, self-statements, and attention-diversion—which are further divided into a total of 10 subcategories.[19] He discusses the trimodal system of pain management: (1) cognitive strategies, which involve thoughts, cognitions, and private events that are self-initiated; (2) behavioral manipulation, involving actions, behaviors, and events that are externally manipulated; and (3) physical intervention, which directly involves the body, completely under external control. The first point of entry is the mind, the second is behavior, and the third is the body; these three interactions are completely different.

Pharmacologic management

Stimmel provides a concise review of the pharmacological management of pain.[68] In listing the factors involving inadequate physician prescription of analgesics, Stimmel notes the four common reasons: (1) lack of knowledge of pharmacologic actions, (2) fear of initiating or perpetuating addiction, (3) use of customary and common patterns of drug-prescribing behavior, and (4) development of a power struggle between physician and patient.

Stimmel also provides a step-by-step approach to the patient who complains of pain, with the use of pharmacologic agents. He suggests identifying the source of pain and factors affecting pain threshold and psychological and other factors affecting pain. He then suggests selecting the appropriate analgesic with lowest adverse effect potential that provides effective relief and suggests considering equianalgesic doses when changing medication. He also cautions physicians to prescribe in accordance with analgesic pharmacologic actions and for sufficient time and in sufficient dose to allow for adequate trial and to use it on a regular basis.[68] He emphasizes that physicians should be aware of untoward side effects—sedation produced by drugs, development of dependence, tolerance, and withdrawal—and recognize that placebo response does not necessarily indicate nonorganic pain and advises physicians to recognize their own bias. The reader is referred to this article and other publications by Stimmel for further review in proper use of pharmacological management of pain problems.[68]

Of the two significant developments in pharmacological management are the development of patient controlled analgesia (PCA) and the use of newer classes of drugs, not usually considered "analgesics." These include predominantly the tricyclic antidepressants, anticonvulsants, psychotropic drugs, and antihistamines.[2, 18, 27, 31, 55, 56, 78] Patient controlled analgesia evolved in response to the inadequacy of intramuscular dosing of narcotic medications. PCA, or "demand analgesia," represents a major advance in the treatment of perioperative pain. Bennett and Griffen review the rationale, technique, safety benefits, and limitation of PCA.[2] PCA also permits individualized analgesic therapy for the patient with chronic cancer pain. Its role in chronic benign pain syndrome has not been explored.

Antidepressants and other "analgesic" drugs

Antidepressants have increasingly been used to treat patients with chronic pain.[9, 18, 27, 31, 43, 55, 56, 68, 74, 78] Although there is association between pain and depression and some authors have classified pain as a masked or atypical depression or even depressive equivalent, there is still dispute whether the drugs exert their influences via analgesic or antidepressant pathways.[18]

A major feature of many of these centrally active drugs is their relative lack of pharmacological specificity. Drugs with anticonvulsant properties, such as carbamazepine (Tegretol), which has the same tricyclic nucleous as Imipramine, are found to have analgesic properties specific for trigeminal neuralgia. The literature is replete with studies of successful use of tricyclic antidepressants such as Imipramine and chlorpramine as analgesics in man. Some authors have postulated a possible similar biochemical similarity between clinical pain and depression.[18] The discovery of endogenous polypetides such as Met-enkephaline and the endorphins possessing "natural" analgesic activity has prompted some authors to argue that both pain and depression are chemically linked. Sternbach has suggested that chronic pain alters the level of brain neurotransmitters and has proposed that inhibition of pain depends on favorable levels of circulating brain serotonin, and perhaps dopamine, and that chronic pain depletes the levels of brain serotonin, particularly in the area of dorsal raphae nucleous. This depletion is thought to account for the apparent ineffectiveness of opiates for analgesia in chronic pain, the apparent increase in pain with chronicity, the association with depression, and the ability of tricyclic antidepressant to reverse symptoms.[66]

Pain relief has been associated either with or without relief of depressive symptoms. Feinmann provides an excellent review of the possible modes of actions of antidepressants in pain management and reviews several current studies available. The conclusion is that there is evidence that tricyclic antidepressants do provide pain relief. The three possible explanations proposed by Feinmann include:[18]

1. Antidepressant agents may alleviate the depressive symptoms associated with or consequent upon chronic suffering, an explanation supported by the several studies. Antidepressants are powerful anesthetics and it is possible that they may also have an anticonvulsant effect due to suppression of neuronal firing, which may contribute to the analgesic effect.
2. There may be a common biochemical mechanism underlying both depression and pain. Thus, Sternbach has suggested that low brain serotonin may lead to hypersensitivity to pain and depression. Pain perception can be reduced by giving serotonin precursers such as L-tryptophan, which also potentiates endogenous opiates, whereas pain, which lowers both noradrenaline and serotonin in the brain, increases pain awareness and accelerates tolerance to morphine. Tricyclics have been shown to inhibit neuronal uptake and increase synaptic serotonin, noradrenaline, and dopamine.
3. The naturally occurring endorphines and enkephalins may be involved. The same brain amines have been shown to have either positive or negative modulatory effects on analgesic activity of morphine—thus, the potentiation of serotonin availability where antidepressants may be sufficient to boost the action of endogenous opiates and to relieve the perception of pain. Thus, Feinmann concludes, pain relief obtained with tricyclic antidepressants is independent of antidepressant effect and the medication must be maintained for three to six months to prevent relapse. Further long-term studies are necessary to support these findings.

Goldenberg and associates, in a randomized, controlled trial of amitriptyline and naproxen in patients with fibromyalgia, noticed that amitriptyline was associated with significant improvement in all outcome parameters including patient and physician global assessment, patient's pain, sleep difficulties, fatigue on awakening, and tender point score.[27] The authors conclude that amitriptyline or amitriptyline with naproxen is an effective therapeutic regimen for patients with fibromyalgia.[27] These authors also reviewed the variety of other studies in the use of tricyclic antidepressants and nonsteroidal inflammatory drugs in the management of a variety of chronic pain states.

In a study of Carette and associates, however, amitriptyline was evaluated in primary fibrositis using the double-blind placebo controlled study. The amitriptyline group improved significantly with respect to sleep patterns and patient and physician global assessment.[9] At low doses, amitriptyline has predominantly hypnotic properties, causing REM suppression and prolongation of stages 3 and 4 non-REM sleep. The alteration of sleep pattern observed in patients with fibrositis is corrected by amitriptyline and may be the major effect of these medications. However, in Carette's study, although there was significant relief of symptoms of fibrositis, there was little effect on fibrositic point tenderness.[9]

Rosenblatt and associates review the use of tricyclic antidepressants in the treatment of depression and chronic pain and provide supporting evidence.[55] They noted that tricyclic antidepressants blocked the histamine H-1 receptors, and more recent studies show a similar blockade of histamine H-2 receptors. Thus, antidepressants have also been used in peptic ulcer disease and pain. The authors conclude that tricyclic antidepressants are superior to alternate modes of therapy when compared in terms of efficacy and risks and the use of tricyclic antidepressants, whether given alone or in conjunction with other drugs, represents a major advance in the present state of care for the patient with chronic pain.[55]

Urban and co-workers have used antidepressant medication with methadone.[74] A combination of a serotonergic reuptake blocking agent and a narcotic was found to be successful in modulating chronic pain. Methadone, 10mg to 20mg daily, and an antidepressant, 25mg to 150mg daily; are more frequently used. Medication is used on a time-contingent basis and in conjunction with other pain rehabilitation approaches. Urban and colleagues report the use of the methadone and antidepressant combination with patients with phantom limb pain. They emphasize the low addictive potential of methadone, the low daily dose, time-contingent administration, and proper patient selection as key factors showing success with their group of patients.[74]

Ward reviews the role of tricyclic antidepressant for chronic low back pain and the mechanisms of action and predictors of response.[78] The author reports strong data to support a serotonergic mechanism of action for antidepressants. The analysis indicates no significant effect of antidepressants on the endogenous opiate systems. The anxiety–muscle tension hypothesis for tricyclic antidepressant was not supported by the data. Similarly, the analysis failed to support the "masked depression" or pain as a "depressive equivalent" hypothesis.[78]

Gurely and co-workers report a controlled study of a serotonin reuptake blocker, zimeladine, in treatment of chronic pain.[31] Zimeladine inhibits the central neuronal reuptake of serotonin to a much greater extent when compared to its effect on nonadrenaline reuptake. The authors quote several clinical studies showing that zimeladine is as effective as amitriptyline, clomipramine, and desipramine in the treatment of depression. They also note that zimeladine was shown to be more effective than placebo treatment of pain syndromes. They used a double-blind crossover study comparing zimeladine with placebo in patients with chronic benign pain. They noted that global assessment of its effectiveness revealed a significant difference in the favor of pain relieving effect of zimeladine when compared to placebo based on physician rating but not patient rating. The authors conclude that serotonin reuptake blockers may have an advantage over other antidepressant drugs with respect to low incidence in severity of side effects.[31]

Watson and Evans report on a comparative trial of amitriptyline and zimeladine in postherpetic neuralgia. They concluded that amitriptyline has pain-relieving action, at least in postherpetic neuralgia, which was not primarily linked with serotonergic effects and also independent of its effect on depression.[79] In patients who did not improve with zimeladine, amitriptyline subsequently resulted in good to excellent response. The authors feel that their study "cast out" serotonergic action of tricyclics in relieving pain.[79] Antidepressants in low doses (25 mg to 50 mg a day) may be of benefit both to depressed and nondepressed patients in potentiating the effects of prescribed analgesics. Patients with endogenous depression may require a dose of 150 mg to 200 mg a day, continued for six months or longer. Despite the frequent use of antidepressants in chronic pain, their mechanism action is unknown.[57]

There does not appear to be any significant difference between one antidepressant versus the other. In certain painful neuropathies and postherpetic neuralgia, however, the patient may benefit from an antidepressant combined with a major tranquilizer—for example, amitriptyline (Elavil, Endep) 25 mg to 100 mg at bedtime combined with perphenzine (Trilafon), 4 mg to 8 mg a day or fluphenazine (Permatil, Prolixin), 1 mg to 6 mg a day, either tranquilizer in divided doses.[57,68]

Walsh and co-workers studied the analgesic effects of D-phenylanine, which is shown to increase the pain thresholds in animals. D-phenylanine (DPA) has been used in studies and has shown a response rate of 32 percent to 75 percent in improving patients with chronic pain. However, the study by Walsh and co-workers did not show any significant analgesic effect from DPA in chronic pain patients when compared to placebo.[77]

Mendel and co-workers have used amitriptyline and fluphenazine in the treatment of painful diabetic neuropathy using a double-blind placebo-controlled, crossover study. This was a study with only six diabetic patients. The researchers noticed only a placebo response with no additional effect of amitriptyline and fluphenazine. As these medications can cause significant side effects, and because the natural course of painful diabetic neuropathy is variable and the perception of pain is so responsive to placebos, the authors caution the use of these medications.[43] The authors emphasize, however, that amitriptyline and Imipramine have both been shown to be superior to placebos in the treatment of painful diabetic neuropathy when it is associated with depression.

Schott and Loh recently described the use of anticholinesterase drugs in the treatment of chronic pain. Both short-acting parenteral and oral anticholinesterase preparations were employed with relief in patients with chronic pain; the authors emphasize that this may be new and potentially valuable approach to treatment of chronic pain. This study was on three patients with central pain.[58] Rumore and Schlichting reviewed the efficacy of antihistamines as analgesics.[56] Histamine is an essential neurotransmitter or neuromodulator. The review indicates direct analgesic effects of various antihistamines. Diphenhydramine, hydroxyzine, or orphandrine, and pyrimaline have been shown to produce analgesia simple entities. Orphandrine and phenyltoloxamane have shown adjuvant effects with acedomedaphin and aspirin.[56] The mechanisms of action remain speculative, but this is an area of potential research.

Results of pain rehabilitation programs

The last 10 years have seen an explosion in the literature of results from a variety of pain facilities. Swanson and co-workers reported the experience of their program from the Mayo Clinic. This was an inpatient program intended to help the patient and family cope with pain, to teach self-treatment methods, and, if possible, to reduce pain. Treatment included behavior modification, physical measures, medication management, and family member participation. Behavior modification emphasized alteration of pain behaviors, increase in physical activities, and reinforcement of improved function. The other measures included education, group and individual exercises, development of work-related activities, and self-administered physical and occupational therapy modalities such as heat and electrical stimulation. Medication management included elimination of all pain-related medications, gradual change of medications to nonaddictive medication, and use of psychotropic medications. Family member participation consisted of involvement of spouse or other important family members in the program, discussions of the patient's pain problem and effect on the family and instruction and application of operant approaches, and use of medication and review of family communication. The other psychological approaches included group discussions of pain-related topics with videotaped demonstrations, biofeedback-assisted relaxation techniques, and supportive treatment. All patients admitted to the program had a complete medical evaluation, a pain problem of six months duration or longer, no related malignant disease, no specific medical or surgical treatment applicable, and acceptance by the patient of the treatment regimen.[70]

The Mayo Clinic population initially consisted of 50 patients between 1974 and 1975. The typical patient had pain in the low back and leg for seven years with a half dozen hospitalizations, two surgical procedures, various other treatments, all of which failed, had not worked for two years, and was receiving compensation. Moderate to marked overall improvement was noted in 54 percent of admitted patients, with failure group including a third of the patients, who left the program early. The program was least successful in reducing subjective pain levels. Greatest success was evident in modifying patient's communication of pain behaviors to others. At a three-and six-month short-term follow-up the number of patients with improvement had decreased from 70 percent to 50 percent; approximately 15 percent to 24 percent had gradual improved functioning after dismissal. The authors conclude that half of the chronically disabled patients who completed the program were able to return home and increase their work-related activity without taking more drugs or returning to the pattern of frequent visits to physician and repeated hospitalization.[70]

Seres and Newman reported the results of treatment from the Portland Pain Center.[61] An inpatient treatment of 21 days duration, the program emphasized operant conditioning, involvement of the spouse, exercise, biofeedback therapy, relaxation therapy, education, use of transcutaneous nerve stimulation, and psychotherapy. Patients reduced medication, increased activity levels, and changed their pain behavior. The authors note, however, that there was little control of patients once they had been discharged from the program.[61] Since this original study, the authors have reported favorable results with an outpatient setting.

Moore and co-workers reported on an inpatient treatment with small group effects in patients with chronic pain. Prior to the program 76.5 percent of the group had been unemployed because of pain and at six-month follow-up this rate had dropped to 55.1 percent. Before treatment only 5.9 percent were fully employed, 14.3 percent after treatment, and 8.2 percent were looking for work or retraining at follow-up.[45]

One of the interesting findings of Moore's study was the relationship of treatment outcome to the structure of the social relationship within which the patient received treatment. Patients who were members of a group in which others failed to respond to a treatment were less likely to benefit from the program. Losing was infectious.[46] Thus it appears that group interaction appears to have a major impact on the treatment course of the individual patient.[46, 71] Moore and co-workers thus suggest that it may be reasonable to "plant" individuals who have successfully responded to previous inpatient treatment program into new groups. Such a positive role model might enhance positive group influence. In analyzing the cost of using "previous winners or spouses" in inpatient treatment programs, they noted "it may actually be a saving to society, in one case would exceed $400,000".[45]

Gottlieb and co-workers report a comprehensive rehabilitation of patients with chronic low back pain. Of the 72 patients treated, 57 demonstrated unimpaired physical functioning and 59 were vocationally restored.[28]

Vasudevan and co-workers report on an outpatient program for managing patients with chronic pain.[76] Seventy-eight patients participated in a structured, intensive, and multidisciplinary rehabilitation program. There were significant improvements in medication reduction and return to work. The authors conclude that outpatient management may be cost-effective management, but for patients with significant medication abuse/dependence, excessive pain behavior, and residence a long distance from treatment facility, a structured inpatient pain rehabilitation program with generalization techniques would be more appropriate.[76]

Jarvikoski and co-workers emphasize that with those outpatients showing high levels of psychological distress, environmental and work stresses persisting during the treatment, may reduce their capacity to benefit from the intervention. On the other hand, outpatient treatment seemed very suitable for those who had back pain as their only health problem and were not deeply distressed by it or by environmental stress factors. Their study also pointed that the inpatient treatment showed a greater variety of positive treatment effects. This kind of treatment can, then, be suitable for those patients who need at least temporary relief from their stressful situation before being mentally or physically able to adopt and take further advantage of the back treatment. Inpatient treatment is particularly appropriate for those who are not able or willing to analyze the cognitive schemas and emotions connected to their illness as a standard practice in multimodal pain centers.[35] The long-term maintenance of treatment benefits will require a long-term outpatient continuation of the changes in behavior and skills learned during the inpatient treatment phase.

Chapman and co-workers also conclude that significant improvement occurs in patients with relatively brief outpatient pain rehabilitation programs and that pending or current disabilities are not necessarily an indication of likely treatment failure.[11] The relatively brief outpatient program at relatively low cost was able to accomplish the goals. With the multimodal treatment program, however, Chapman emphasizes that it is impossible to assess which modalities produce which benefits.

A common feature of multidisciplinary pain rehabilitation programs provide patients with (1) an opportunity to play an active role in their treatment, (2) education and information about the pain experience, and (3) the opportunity to interact with other patients with similar problems and find ways of living satisfying lives.

Lutz and co-workers reviewed the treatment outcome and compliance following multidisciplinary pain programs. Compliance with prescribed therapeutic regimens was found to be low, averaging about 42 percent for individual regimens. Only 12.3 percent of the respondents in their study complied with the total combination of prescribed regimens. The authors also point out that "the degree to which daily compliance from multiple therapeutic regimens is actually needed for different types of pain problems is unclear." Lutz and co-workers thus conclude that patient compliance with treatment regimens clearly cannot be taken for granted and that patient regression to pretreatment levels may well be due to insufficient follow-through with the skills and treatments learned and performed while participating in the pain program.[40] This provides an increasingly strong argument for continuing support groups wherein activities are reviewed and support is provided.

Sturgis and co-workers report an important study on results from a pain center of treated and untreated patients.[69] In this group the nontreated group was untreated only in the sense that the patients did not participate in a multidisciplinary rehabilitation program. These patients continued contact with the physician or a health professional. The follow-up study indicates that a number of the untreated patients also reportedly used the same strategies for pain control as the treated subjects. They discovered these techniques through trial-and-error, a finding that lends validity to the inclusion of these techniques in pain rehabilitation programs. The study did show, however, that treated patients were more active in employing nonmedicinal strategies for pain control. In this study, the authors found that even in the treated group, pain-related self-control techniques were limited and the patient typically used only one or two strategies to control pain levels. Continued, active employment of self-control strategies is necessary if the maximum efficiency of the treatment is to be maintained. Sturgis and co-workers thus conclude that treatment effectiveness needs to be evaluated in a more controlled manner and that, in evaluating the cost effectiveness of treatment program, the cost and benefits of alternative treatments need to be examined. They also emphasize the importance of follow-up of patient treatment adherence after discharge.

Guck and co-workers also report on a follow-up study from a multidisciplinary pain center comparing a treatment with a nontreatment control group.[30] The control group members met the admission criteria but were unable to participate in the program because they did not have financial coverage. The four-week inpatient program involved three components: (1) gradual reduction and eventual elimination of all nonnarcotic, narcotic, and psychotropic pain medication using a fixed schedule, (2) progressive increase of daily exercise and physical activity, and (3) identification and resolution of psychosocial issues related to or caused by the pain situation.

At follow-up 60 percent of the treated patients met all criteria for success while none of the untreated patients met these criteria.[29,30] Significantly more treated patients were employed at follow-up than untreated patients. In addition, treated patients reported less pain-related interference with work, household chores, yardwork and shopping, socialization, hobbies and recreational activities, sexual relationships, physical exercise, and ability to sleep than did the untreated group. Treated patients also reported more "up time," lower pain levels, and less depression than untreated patients.[29] Similarly, the treated group was hospitalized significantly less often at follow-up than the untreated group. Fewer treated than nontreated patients were using prescription narcotics and psychotropic medications after treatment. An interesting finding was that there was no difference in the number of treated and untreated patients using nonnarcotic medications at follow-up.[29,30]

Guck and co-workers also found no difference between the groups in number of individuals receiving compensation or with pending litigation. The study had several positive features including the fact that most of the information was not obtained on self-report questionnaires but rather from hospital records on employment status, compensation, and litigation. The response rate was high for both treated and untreated patients, thus providing a representative sample. A diversity of outcome criteria, including the use of the health care system, subjective pain levels, and depression scores, was used in this study. Taken together, the results of the study by Guck and co-workers indeed indicate that individuals treated at multidisciplinary pain centers return to a more normal, less disabled lifestyle significantly more often than untreated patients.[29,30]

Factors affecting outcome

Guck and co-workers report on predicting long-term outcome of multidisciplinary pain treatment.[29] The results of this study demonstrated that successfully treated patients were (1) less likely to be receiving compensation, (2) younger, (3) less likely to be taking psychotropic medications, and (4) had undergone fewer pretreatment pain-related surgeries than unsuccessfully treated patients.

Drug use and the number of pain surgeries have emerged as predictive factors in previous studies. In Guck's study only the use of psychotropic medication appeared in the prediction equation. However, other medication-related variables, including the use of nonnarcotics and narcotics, shared a considerable amount of variance with psychotropic medication so that in general it can be said that pretreatment use of medication (along with the number of pain-related surgeries) appears to have bearing on the prediction of follow-up outcome.[29] Age, compensation, and education did not have a significant relationship with outcome but made significant and unique contributions to the classification equations in Guck's study.[29]

At this time there do not appear to be any clear predictors for use as entry criteria for multidisciplinary pain programs. Obviously, if ideal patients are selected using very stringent criteria, the success rate could definitely improve. However, identifying who will benefit from treatment or from particular nonsurgical treatment needs further elucidation.

Maruta and co-workers, in attempting to identify those patients who benefit from a pain management program, studied a group that did well at one year follow-up as opposed to a group that failed. The factors that differed significantly between the groups included duration of pain, work time lost, number of operations, subjective pain relief, and drug dependency. The seven-item rating scale based on these data differentiated a favorable group from the unfavorable group.[42]

Pain of less than three years duration and work time lost of less than one year were favorable indicators, whereas pain of five years duration or more and work time lost of 1.5 years or more were unfavorable indicators. The number of operations related to pain was significantly higher in the failure group, with one or less operations being a favorable indicator and three or more operations being an unfavorable indicator. Pain levels of 5 or less were favorable whereas pain levels of 7 more were unfavorable. Significantly higher drug dependency was found in the failure group, an unfavorable indicator. Different elevations of hypochondriasis and hysteria scales on an MMPI also seem to differentiate the two groups.[42]

Hamburgen used the same seven-item scale used by Maruta and co-workers and report that it was not a clinically useful predictor of treatment success.[33] The correlation between loss of work time and outcome was significant only at follow-up. High pain level was one of the most useful items in identifying patients unlikely to succeed in the program.

Crook compared the persistent pain suffers in a specialty pain clinic with those in the community. One group was drawn from a "typical family medical practice" and the other from a "specialized multidisciplinary pain clinic." The two groups were similar in most demographic variables, the length of pain history, and the most common reported sites of pain. However, patients from the pain clinic were more likely to have had work-related accidents, to report greater health care utilization, and to complain of more constant pain and greater levels of disability. Patients from the pain clinic also reported a greater impairment on the indices constructed to measure psychological, social, and performance consequences of the pain experience. What most distinguished patients from the pain clinic was not the medical factors alone, but reported impairment that reflected in daily function and psychosocial difficulties. The authors conclude that the patients referred to specialized pain clinics may not be representative of individuals in general who suffer persistent pain, the former likely requiring an interdisciplinary approach that includes attention to psychosocial disability issues and not just medical or surgical treatment of pain.[12]

Crook and co-workers thus conclude that it is likely that patients referred to chronic pain clinics are not representative of individuals, in general, who suffer persistent pain and it would therefore be unwise to make generalizations about chronic pain clinic patients that would equate them with all pain sufferers. The authors emphasize that chronic pain does not mean pain beyond six months but the psychosocial distress that increases the probability of the patient being referred to a chronic pain clinic.[12]

Linton provides the most current review on the behavioral remediation of chronic pain.[38] A major problem with the reported studies is the long-term effects of such treatment. There are problems in methodology of these studies, including low return rates, the use of global ratings and questionnaires, and non-blind collection of data. Linton notes that if one considers the variable of returning to work, most of the successful studies report one-year rates of approximately 50 percent. Thus he emphasizes that complete rehabilitation for all patients is, at this time, an unrealistic goal.[38] Thus in those where return to work is not possible, treatment should be oriented toward helping the patient live as normally and productively as possible. A second alternative is to prevent the development of chronic pain.[38]

Pain and litigation

Patients with chronic pain are the primary source of information regarding their pain. Thus the opportunity for malingering—that is, the deliberate faking of symptoms for the sole purpose of obtaining an extrinsic goal—is ever present. Leavitt and Sweet recently studied the characteristics and frequency of malingering among patients with low back pain. They reviewed 150 board-certified neurosurgeons and 150 board-certified orthopedic surgeons to identify factors related to malingering. Perception in the magnitude of malingering ranges from a low of 1 percent to a high of 75 percent. However, the estimates were not evenly spread, and approximately 40 percent of physicians, estimates were in the range of 1 percent to 2 percent. Of the criteria rated as important to identify malingering by the physician were:

1. Pain that does not follow an organic pattern.
2. Endorsement of false symptom suggestion.
3. Cogwheel weakness.

4. Overreaction during examination.

Interestingly, pending litigation was seen as important only by half of the sample, and financial compensation was rated as important by only 35 percent.[37] This survey had a return rate of only 38.3 percent. It should be noted that it is common for patients with low back pain and psychological disturbance to overreact during examination, to show patterns of pain that do not follow organic patterns, and to display levels of disability that far exceed that which can be justified on the basis of objective findings. Thus, frequently multidimensional syndromes may be mistakenly diagnosed as malingering.[37]

Dworkin and associates, studying the relationship between compensation, litigation, and employment on the treatment response to the patient with chronic pain, not that there is indeed a relationship between treatment response and compensation and litigation. The results of long-term outcome were consistent with the short-term outcome. Compensation benefits and unemployment status both predicted poor short-term outcome; however, when employment and compensation were jointly used to predict outcome, only employment was significant. The authors conclude that it is important to redirect patients from the deleterious effects of the "compensation neurosis and towards roles of activity and employment in the treatment and rehabilitation of chronic pain patients."[15,16]

Patients with pain and litigation pending present a high-risk group for treatment. However, the studies of the past several years reveal inconsistent findings. Trief and Stein, in their study of patients with litigation and rehabilitation outcome of chronic back pain, found that immediate beneficial effects of treatment were significantly less for the group with litigation pending. This was evidenced on the MMPI as well as by behavioral measures of physical mobility. Both groups significantly improved from the treatment; however, the no-litigation group improved at a relatively faster rate and the improvement level remain stable throughout a one- and three-month follow-up. Thus, they recommend not withholding treatment from those individuals until litigation is resolved.[73] Similarly, Reynolds and co-workers found the use of transcutaneous electrical nerve stimulation not to be any less effective where patients had possible secondary gain motives. The lack of association was felt probably related to differences in patients' perception of treatment goals. While some treatments such as surgery and nerve blocks were offered to the chronic pain patient to permanently eliminate pain, TENS is usually prescribed to control otherwise intractable pain.[53]

Assessment of pain and the results of treatment

Aronoff et al. review the follow-up studies of multidisciplinary pain units. The reviews from many centers indicate varying results. The authors note a lack of any standardized assessment procedure, therefore making it impossible to compare effectiveness of treatment programs or various comparison groups.[1] These authors suggest possible tests such as McGill-Melzack Pain Questionnaire, Profile of Mood States or other tests of depression and mood, the Pilowsky Illness Behaviour Questionnaire, and the Sickness Impact Profile. Further tests of vocational and avocational activities along with standardized physical activities and social functioning would have to be found or developed. In addressing the difficulty of finding control groups the author suggests the following: First, one could compare persons who complete the program with those who leave against medical advice or are judged to be unsatisfactory in their participation in the programs—those who have not received treatment for technical reasons such as lack of insurance coverage or are rejected from treatment as inappropriate. Second, one could use a waiting list control group. The authors point to the difficulty of finding patients who are acceptable for treatment and probably would successfully participate in a pain unit program but do not, an almost impossible task. Another problem to consider, the authors note, is that when comparing data from various pain units, each program varies from its medical orientation, type of treatments, length of treatments, and so on.[1]

Several studies in the literature continue to report "improvement" with chronic pain rehabilitation programs despite the lack of uniform criteria to measure success. They point that behavioral methods do *not* have as their principal objective the modification of nocioception nor the direct modification of the experience of pain, although, as frequently happens, both are influenced by these methods[20, 21, 22] Rather, *behavioral methods* in pain treatment programs *are intended to treat excess disability and expression of suffering*. This is done by changing the relationship between these behaviors and the reinforcing contingencies and thus the goal is to render the chronic pain patient more functional and as normal in behavior as possible. Thus, the alteration of social contingencies plays the primary role in bringing about the changes in patients with chronic pain. "Normality" is defined by several authors using the following criteria at the time of follow-up:[22, 23]

1. Males must have been employed unless they are retired,
2. Retired males must have functioned to their own and their family's satisfaction and be physically active eight hours or more a day,
3. Women must have been employed if necessary for their own or their children's support,
4. Married women not gainfully employed must have been functioning to their own and their family's satisfaction and be physically active at least eight hours or more a day,
5. The patient must not have been receiving any compensation whether employed or not,
6. The patient must not have had any pain-related hospitalization since discharge from the treatment program,
7. The patient must not have been using any prescription analgesics, sedatives, muscle relaxants, or tranquilizers.

Heaton and co-workers, in an attempt to assess chronic pain with its multiple psychosocial factors, developed an evaluation system called the Psychosocial Pain Inventory.[34] Scores on the PSPI were approximately normally distributed and had good interrater reliability. Patients with high PSPI scores were more likely to be considered as exaggerating their symptoms during physical examination, but they did not show less evidence of an organic basis for pain. Significant correlations obtained between PSPI scores and some measures from the McGill Pain Questionnaire but were essentially unrelated to personality disturbances as measured by the MMPI. The PSPI and the MMPI seem to provide different types of information that can be used in a complementary way in evaluating pain patients. High scores on the PSPI predict poor response to medical treatment for pain.[34]

Doleys and co-workers note that self-reported pain intensities are frequently used measures for chronic pain. Patients are frequently used to rate their pain on a 0 to 10 or similar lichert scale. The authors also note that the effects of narcotics on pain ratings have not been well controlled especially in self-reported pain ratings between those who use narcotics and nonnarcotics. Doleys and co-workers emphasize that there is a statistically significant decrease in self-reported pain ratings between the time of evaluation and the beginning of treatment.[14] They feel that the change might reflect inflated ratings at evaluation, decreased anxiety secondary to acceptance into the treatment program, decreased ratings as a funtion of being in the treatment setting, and expectation for change. Thus, it is clear that pain ratings obtained during evaluation should not be considered the most accurate pretreatment ratings.[14] They also noted that the magnitude and rate of decrease in pain ratings during treatment were greater than those between evaluation and pretreatment. They conclude that the passage of time could not completely account for the observed changes. They note, however, that the regular narcotic users showed a slower rate of decreasing patterns in self-reported pain and a smaller degree of change during treatment than did the groups not using narcotics. The posttreatment ratings of regular users may reflect a difference in pain perception with and without the influence of narcotis more than the effect of treatment.[14]

Doleys' data have significant implication for assessing treatment effectiveness. Instead of a criteria of no increase in self-reported pain as suggested by some authors, a minimum 10 percent decrease in self-reported pain should be expected to occur on an average.[14]

Fordyce and co-workers recently reviewed the approaches used in pain measurement and pain behavior.[22] They found a positive relationship between patient-generated statements about severity of pain and extent of functional impairment from pain. However, these measures showed few relationships to medication consumption, health care utilization, daily recorded activity level, or patient-reported frequency counts of engaging in a set of commonplace activities.[22] Thus, there is a question of relationship between what people say about their pain and what they do. Accordingly, the evaluation of chronic pain should include analysis of patient behavior rather than patient rating of pain severity.

Patient's ratings about severity of associated impairments and series of behavioral measures of health care utilization and activity patterns should be used as measures.

The measurement of clinical pain is essential to the evalution of pain problems and treatment effects. However, little consensus regarding the most appropriate measurement methods is present. There does not appear, however, to be any relationship between what people *say* about their pain—in the form of magnitude estimates—and their behavior. The results display little or no relationship. Yet patients' ratings of severity of pain and claimed amount of activity and limitations were significantly related. However, those pain and claimed impairment ratings, when analyzed against patient-recorded frequencies and the amount of health care utilization, medication consumption, body position, and time or frequency of engaging in commonplace activities, fail to show consistent relationships. These findings further support the conceptual point that pain behaviors (that is, how pain/suffering is communicated) have significance in their own right. The behaviors of pain patients may diverge according to a variety of factors not necessarily associated with the nature of the body damage from which the pain problems arose. The direct observation of behavior clearly would be a preferred method. Direct measurement of amount of time a person sits, reclines, stands, and walks, obtained from observers following the person around, makes appropriate recordings. Perhaps a time sampling basis would presumably yield the greatest validity. Fordyce concludes that reported frequencies of activities may be a more closely related measure of "actual" activity than our ratings or statements about the extent to which activities are curtailed by pain.[22]

Gatchel and co-workers described the use of the Millon Behavioral Health Inventory (MBHI) in predicting physical function in patients with low back pain.[25] These authors also note that physical findings frequently do not correlate well with self-reported pain symptoms in patients with chronic pain. The Millon Behavioral Health Inventory was used as a major psychological assessment device. This 150 item self-report inventory was orginally developed for psychological assessment of individuals undergoing evaluation for treatment for physical disorders in medical settings. Unlike the MMPI, originally designed for a psychiatric population, the MBHI was developed and standardized on a medical population. The change in the MBHI scales from admission to follow-up assessment was used as a predictor variable. The absolute admission MBHI scores do not show significant predictive relationship, but some of the subsets do. The authors conclude that the clinical use of the MBHI in predicting improvement in physical functioning and adherence to treatment program in chronic low back pain is a real possibility.[25]

Ready and co-workers compared self-reported versus actual use of medications in the chronic pain patient population and note that patients with chronic pain tend to underestimate their medication use and that this tendency is greater for narcotic analgesics than for a variety of other medications taken for pain.[52] Their findings suggest that when drug problems are identified or suspected, objective information about drug use should be obtained before attempting to regulate it or to diagnose and treat an underlying pain problem. They recommend expressing dosage in terms of drug equivalants in comparing medication use among patients.[51]

Schwartz and co-workers studied the assessment of beliefs and attitudes of chronic pain patients by use of a brief psychoeducatinal videotape and questionnaire. Patient attitudes and belief about information relevant to appropriate treatment can be reliably assessed by their reactions to a psychoeducational videotape. The authors conclude that the responses to the videotape can serve as a "red flag" to indicate patient-clinic misunderstanding or miscommunication.[60]

Toomey and co-workers emphasized the need of multiple functional criteria in assessing response to treatment including both global pain ratings and functional-behavioral measures of improvement.[72] Functional-behavioral measures include downtime, ability to bend and walk, work ability, recreational and social abilities, health-seeking behaviors, and frequency and intensity of pain. Isolated criteria for pain reduction and return to work are too narrow for assessment of patient outcome.

Prevention of chronic pain

Prevention of chronic pain syndrome would be ideal. Is chronic pain preventable? Oosterhuis emphasizes that early screening of pain may prevent pain from becoming intractable.[48] He reviews the literature and indicates that "the general practitioner knows how to cope with 95 percent of the pain problems, either by eliminating the cause or because the pain is self limited." He discusses the common dilemma faced by physicians. On the one hand the general practitioner must not deny patients timely intervention in cases of possibly serious diseases, while on the other hand the practitioner should not let those who have no disease at all run the risk of becoming chronic complainers.[48] He provides several examples and concludes:

> Giving the patient an insight into the relationship between his pain and the painful situation may in itself be therapeutic, even when the doctor cannot always change circumstances for his patients. To attribute the pain to stressful circumstances and not the disease may help to give the patient a grip on his situation and may lessen the anxiety that may arise from being helpless and dependent on doctors to end the pain. In the meantime it may be useful—to keep open the possibility of discussing the painful problem—to engage the assistance of other professional.[48]

In a presentation titled "Chronic Pain: Is It Necessary?" Rene Cailliet discusses the burden of pain on the health care system and points to the tunnel vision of specialists in dealing with pain based on their particular domain.[8] Before the chronic phase occurs, an acute phase must logically exist in the sequence of pain perception. He reviews the conceptual model proposed by Loeser which includes: (1) *nocioception*, the tissue irritation at the peripheral site of injury or disease, which may be thermal, chemical, mechanical, or electrical; (2) *pain*, indicating transmission within neural pathways of the nervous system, both peripheral and central; (3) *suffering*, which is the affective response to pain influenced by experience and emotions, which may or may not be related to nocioceptive stimuli or to pain; and finally (4) *pain behavior*, which is expressed by the sufferer, witnessed by society, accepted by peers, and expresses a request for a specific response by society.[8]

Suffering and pain behavior are the actions that permit the sufferer to enter the health care delivery system. All the four components need not to be evident or in the sequence noted, but frequently they are. Thus, Cailliet emphasizes that interruption of the sequence offers hope of modifying the ultimate behavior.[8] Interrupting or modifying the nocioceptive pain may influence progression before a chronic engram is indelibly imprinted upon the central nervous system. He rightfully emphasizes that "physicians too frequently remain the therapist rather than the teacher."[8]

Chronic pain patients, as a group, are generally viewed as being either neurotic or having a "pain prone personality."[17] Murphy and Cornish attempted to predict chronicity in a group of patients with acute low back pain.[46] Patients presenting with complaints of low back pain of less than six months duration and seen for the first time were studied. Six months after the initial contact all subjects received a follow-up questionnaire, and the factors predicting the chronicity were then reviewed. The authors were able to identify 24 out of 27 prechronic cases as chronic, for a hit rate of 85.7 percent.[46] In general, a prechronic pain patient had the following features: (1) complains of pain at numerous body sites, (2) more often has deep musculoskeletal rather than peripheral pain, (3) is highly anxious in the acute stage, and (4) does not have any activity level sufficient to preclude a preoccupation with pain. The useful aspect of the study is to identify which of the many variables are most promising for future research and to intervene during the acute stage before the patient reaches the point of needing a pain clinic. Thus, several authors believe that if acute pain is managed effectively, chronic pain can possibly be prevented.

CONCLUSIONS

Chronic pain, in addition to being a complex phenomenon, is a major health and social problem taxing the health care resources and causing economic burden to society. There have been significant advances in the understanding and management of patients with chronic pain. These major developments are the differentation between acute and chronic pain, the recognition of the role of learning and operant conditioning genesis of chronic pain behaviors, and the relationship of cognition and behavior factors in chronic pain states.

The major emphasis in providing care for these patients and families is in a pain center, a facility that has a multidisciplinary team of physician, social worker, vocational rehabilitation counselors, and so on. These centers provide an outpatient evaluation and then treatment in either an inpatient or outpatient setting or a combination or variations of these. Reports of such treatment programs that use a combination of approaches and techniques indicate that the patients reveal improvement in several parameters. Inpatient programs seem best suited to provide a structured environment, one indicated in patients with drug dependence/abuse, significant physical deconditioning requiring supervised graded activities, excessive pain behaviors requiring a structured group milieu operant conditioning, and those whose living arrangements are not conducive for access of an outpatient facility. Outpatient programs are generally less expensive, provide a "natural and real" environment, make generalization of learned techniques easier, and assist in breaking the "sick role" associated with hospitalizations.

Chronic pain syndromes that do not have significant psychosocial alterations can be managed, using techniques based on neurophysiological and neurochemical basis. Such patients are effectively managed in syndrome-oriented clinics, such as specialized headache clinics, temporomandibular joint dysfunction centers, back schools, and nerve block clinics. Although initially available only at large university centers, multidisciplinary rehabilitation programs and syndrome-oriented pain clinics are now becoming available in smaller community hospitals, making accessibility easier.

Although psychological interventions have been the major change in the initial years, the last few years have been characterized by pharmacologic manipulation. The use of antidepressant group of drugs has opened the doors to potentially many more alternatives for drug treatment. This field of neurochemical modulation shows great promise.

The major challenge facing those involved with the management of patients with chronic pain, including physicians, other health care providers and third-party payers, is the need for measures of success effected by the treatments. Accountability and "quality control" of pain centers in the future depends on developing a standardized assessment of treatment program effectiveness that is objective, quantifiable, and reproducible. This is imperative at a time of limited resources. Organizations such as the Commission on Accreditation of Rehabilitation Facilities (CARF) have developed standards in this area.[65] Other chapters in this book address the status and progress being made in these areas.

Although the advances in pain management, like most fields of medicine, have been amoeboid, there has definitely been progress in the understanding and management of the patient with chronic pain. Education of the physician, health care community, and third-party payers and utilization of research developed in the last 25 years should assist in the humane caring of these individuals with chronic pain and suffering in the future.

REFERENCES

1. Aronoff GM, Evans WO, Engers PL: A review of follow up studies of multidisciplinary pain units. Pain 16:1–11, 1983.
2. Bennett RL, Griffen WO: Patient-controlled analgesia (PCA): optimization of inhospital narcotic analgesic therapy. Clin Orth 6(5):67–77, 1983.
3. Benzon HT: Epidural steroid injections for low back pain and lumbosacral radiculopathy. Pain 24: 227–295, 1986.

4. Black RG: The chronic pain syndrome. Surg Clin N Am 55:999–1011, 1975.
5. Bonica JJ: Importance of the problem. In: Aronoff GM, (ed.) Evaluation and Treatment of Chronic Pain. Baltimore: Urban & Schwarzenberg, 1985.
6. Brena SF, Chapman SL: Management of Patients with Chronic Pain. New York: SP Medical and Scientific Books, 1983.
7. Berna SF: Nerve blocks and chronic pain states—an update. Postgrad Med 76(4):77–86, 1985.
8. Cailliet R: Chronic pain: is it necessary? Arch Phy Med Rehab 60:4–7, 1979.
9. Carette S, McCain GA, Bell DA, Fam AG: Evaluation of amitriptyline in primary fibrositis—a double-blind placebo-controlled study. Arth Rheum 29(5):655–659, 1986.
10. Chapman SL, Brena SF: Learned helplessness and responses to nerve blocks in chronic low back pain patients. Pain 14:355–364, 1982.
11. Chapman SL, Brena SF, Bradford LA: Treatment outcome in a chronic pain rehabilitation program. Pain 11:255–268, 1981.
12. Crook J, Tunks E, Rideout E, Browne G: Epidemiologic comparison of persistent pain sufferers in a specialty pain clinic and in the community. Arch Phy Med Rehab 67:451–455, 1986.
13. Crue BL: Multidisciplinary pain treatment programs: current status. J Clin Pain 1:31–38, 1985.
14. Doleys DM, Dolce JJ, Doleys AL, Crocker M, Wolfe SE: Evaluation, narcotics and behavioral treatment influences on pain ratings in chronic pain patients. Arch Phy Med Rehab 67:456–458, 1986.
15. Dworkin RH, Handlin DS, Richlin DM, Brand L, Vannucci C: Unraveling the effects of compensation, litigation and employment on treatment response in chronic pain. Pain 23:49–59, 1985.
16. Dworkin RH, Richlin DM, Handlin DS, Brand L: Predicting treatment response in depressed and non-depressed chronic pain patients. Pain 24:343–353, 1986.
17. Engel GL: "Psychogenic" pain and the pain-prone patient. Amer J Med 26:899–918, 1959.
18. Feinmann C: Pain relief by antidepressants: possible modes of action. Pain 23:1–8, 1985.
19. Fernandez E: A classification system of cognitive coping strategies for pain. Pain 26:141–1151, 1986.
20. Fordyce WE: Behavioral Methods for Chronic Pain and Illness. St. Louis: C.V. Mosby, 1976.
21. Fordyce WE, Roberts AH, Sternbach RA: The behavioral management of chronic pain: a response to critics. Pain 22:113–125, 1985.
22. Fordyce WE, Lansky D, Calsyn DA, Shelton JL, Stolov WC, Rock DL: Pain measurement and pain behavior. Pain 18:53–69, 1984.
23. France RD, Krishnan KRR, Trainor M: Chronic pain and depression. III. Family history study of depression and alcoholism in chronic low back pain patient. Pain 24:185–190, 1986.
24. Gamsa A, Braha RED, Catchlov RFH: The use of structured group therapy sessions in the treatment of chronic pain patients. Pain 22:91–96, 1985.
25. Gatchel RJ, Mayer TG, Capra P, Barnett J, Diamond P: Millon Behavioral Health Inventory: its utility in predicting physical function in patients with low back pain. Arch Phy Med Rehab 67: 878–882, 1986.
26. Gildenberg DL, Devaul RA: The Chronic Pain Patient—Evaluation and Management. New York: Karger, 1985.
27. Goldenberg DL, Felson DT, Dinerman H: A randomized, controlled trial of amitriptyline and naproxen in the treatment of patients with fibromyalgia. Arth Rheum 29(11):1371–1377, 1986.
28. Gottlieb H, Strite LC, Koller R, Madorsky A, Hockersmith V, Kleeman M, Wagner J: Comprehensive rehabilitation of patients having low back pain. Arch Phy Med Rehab 58:101–108, 1977.
29. Guck TP, Meilman PW, Skultety FM, Dowd E: Prediction of long-term outcome of multidisciplinary pain treatment. Arch Phy Med Rehab 67:293–296, 1986.
30. Guck TP, Skultety FM, Meilman PW, Dowd ET: Multidisciplinary pain center follow up study: evaluation with a no-treatment control group. Pain 21:295–3-06, 1985.
31. Gurely GK, Cherry DA, Cousins MJ, Love BL, Graham JR, McLachlin MO: A controlled study of a serotonin reuptake blocker, zimelidine, in the treatment of chronic pain. Pain 25:35–52, 1986.
32. Haley WE, Turner JA, Romano JM: Depression in chronic pain patients: relation to pain, activity and sex differences. Pain 23:337–343, 1985.
33. Hamburgen ME, Jennings CA, Maruta T, Swanson DW: Failure of a predictive scale in identifying patients who may benefit from a pain management program: follow up data. Pain 23: 253–258, 1985.
34. Heaton RK, Getto CJ, Lehman RA, Fordyce WE, Brauer E, Gorban SE: A standardized evaluation of psychosocial factors in chronic pain. Pain 12:165-174, 1982.

35. Jarvikoski A, Hakapaa K, Mellin G: Symptoms and treatment effects with low-bakc pain patients. Pain 25:345–355, 1986.
36. Krishnan KRR, France RD, Pelton S, McCann UD, Davidson, J, Urban BJ: Chronic pain and depression I. Classification of depression in chronic low back pain patients. Pain 22:279–287, 1985.
37. Leavitt F, Sweet JJ: Characteristics and frequency of malingering among patients with low back pain. Pain 25:357–364, 1986.
38. Linton SJ: Behavioral remediation of chronic pain: a status report. Pain 24:125–141, 1986.
39. Linton SJ: The relationship between activity and chronic back pain. Pain 21:289–294, 1985.
40. Lutz RW, Silbert M, Olshan N: Treatment outcome and compliance with therapeutic regimens: long-term followup of a multidisciplinary pain program. Pain 17:301–308, 1983.
41. Margolis RB, Zimny GH, Miller D, Taylor JM: Internists and the chronic pain patient. Pain 20: 151–156, 1984.
42. Maruta T, Swanson DW, Swenson WM: Chronic pain: which patients may a pain management program help? Pain 7:321–329, 1979.
43. Mendel CM, Klein RF, Chappell DA, Dere WH, Gertz BJ, Karam JH, Lavi TN, Grunfeld C: A trial of amitriptyline and fluphenazine in the treatment of painful diabetic neuropathy. JAMA 255 (5):637–639, 1986.
44. Modlin HC: Posttraumatic stress disorder—no longer just for war veterans. Postgrad Med 79(3): 26–44, 1986.
45. Moore ME, Berk SN, Mypaver A: Chronic pain: inpatient treatment with small group effects. Arch Phy Med Rehab 65:356–361, 1984.
46. Murphy KA, Cornish RD: Prediction of chronicity in acute low back pain. Arch Phy Med Rehab 65:334–337, 1984.
47. Muse M: Stress-related, posttraumatic chronic pain syndrome: criteria for diagnosis, and preliminary report on prevalance. Pain 23:295–300, 1985.
48. Oosterhuis WW: Early screening of pain to prevent it from becoming intractable. Pain 20:193–200, 1984.
49. Pilowsky I: Pain and illness behavior: assessment and management. In: Wall and Melzack (eds.) Textbook of Pain. Edinburgh: Churchill Livingstone, 1984.
50. Pinsky JJ: Chronic, intractable, benign pain: a syndrome and its treatment with intensive short-term group psychotherapy. J Human Stress: 17–21, September 1978.
51. Ready LB, Sarkin E, Turner JA: Self-reported vs. actual use of medications in chronic pain patients. Pain 12:285–294, 1982.
52. Reuler JB, Girard De, Nardone DA: The chronic pain syndrome: misconceptions and management. Ann Intern Med 93:588–596, 1980.
53. Reynolds AC, Abram SE, Anderson RA, Vasudevan SV, Lynch NT: Chronic pain therapy with transcutaneous electrical nerve stimulation: predictive value of questionnaire. Arch Phy Med Rehab 64:311–313, 1983.
54. Richardson PH, Vincent CA: Acupuncture for the treatment of pain: a review of evaluative research. Pain 24:15–40, 1986.
55. Rosenblatt RM, Reich J, Dehring D: Tricyclic antidepressants in the treatment of depression and chronic pain: analysis of the supporting evidence. Anesth Analg 63:1025–32, 1984.
56. Rumore MM, Schlichting DA: Clinical efficacy of antihistaminics as analgesics. Pain 25:7–22, 1986.
57. Ruoff GE, Beery GB: Chronic pain—characteristics, assessment and treatment plans. Postgrad Med 78:91–97, 1985.
58. Schott GD, Loh L: Anticholinesterse drugs in the treatment of chronic pain. Pain 20:201–20, 1984.
59. Schottenfeld RS, Cullen MR: Occupation induced posttraumatic stress disorders. Am J Psych 142: 198–202, 1985.
60. Schwartz DP, DeGood DE, Shutty MS: Direct assessment of beliefs and attitudes of chronic pain patients. Arch Phy Med Rehab 66:806–809, 1985.
61. Seres JL, Newman RL: Result of treatment of chronic low back pain at the Portland Pain Center. J Neurosurg 45:32–36, 1976.
62. Shanfield SB, Heiman EM, Cope DN, Jones JR: Pain and the marital relationship: psychiatric distress. Pain 7:343–359, 1979.
63. Skevington SM: Chronic pain and depression: universal or helplessness?. Pain 15:309–317, 1983.
64. Soric R, Devlin M: Transcutaneous electrical nerve stimulation—practical aspects and appli-

cations. Postgrad Med 78(4):101–107, 1985.
65. Standards Manual for Serving People with Disabilities 1986. Commission on Accreditation of Rehabilitation Facilities, Tucson, Arizona.
66. Sternbach RA: The need for an animal model of chronic pain. Pain 2: 2–4, 1976.
67. Sternbach RA: Pain and "hassles" in the United States: findings of the Nuprin Pain Report. Pain 27:69–80, 1986.
68. Stimmel B: Pain, analgesia and addiction: an approach to the pharmacologic management of pain. Clin J Pain, 1:14–22, 1985.
69. Sturgis ET, Schaefer CA, Sikora TL: Pain center followup study of treated and untreated patients. Arch Phy Med Rehab 65:301–303, 1984.
70. Swanson DW, Swenson WM, Maruta T, McPhee MC: 1. Program description and characteristics of patients, 2. Short-term results. Mayo Clinic Proceedings 51:410–408, 409–411, July 1976.
71. Tan SY: Cognitive and cognitive behavioral methods of pain control: a selective review. Pain 12: 201–228, 1982.
72. Toomey TC, Taylor AG, Skelton JA, Carron H: Stability of self-report measures of improvement in chronic pain: a 5 year follow up. Pain 12:273–283, 1982.
73. Trief P. Stein N: Pending litigation and rehabilitation outcome of chronic back pain. Arch Phy Med Rehab 66:95–99, 1985.
74. Urban BJ, France RD, Steinderger EK, Scott DL, Maltbie AA: Long-term use of narcotic/antidepressant medication in the management of phantom limb pain. Pain 24:191–196, 1986.
75. Vasudevan SV, Lynch NT: Counseling the patient with chronic pain—role of the physician. In: Lynch and Vasudevan (eds.) Persistent Pain: Psychosocial Assessment and Intervention. Boston: Martinus Nijhoff.
76. Vasudevan SV, Lynch NT, Grunert BK, Melvin JL, Abram SE: Outpatient management of chronic pain: long term results. Wis Med J 84:7–9, May 1985.
77. Walsh NE, Ramaruthy S, Schoenfeld L, Hoffman J: Analgesic effectiveness of D-Phenylalanine in chronic pain patients. Arch Phy Med Rehab 67:436–439, 1986.
78. Ward NG: Tricyclic antidepressants for chronic low back pain—mechanisms of action and predictors of response. Spine 11(7):661–665, 1986.
79. Watson CPN, Evans RJ: A comparative trial of amitriptyline and zemelidine in post herpeticneur algia. PAIN 23:387–394, 1985.

6. PROBLEMS IN PAIN MANAGEMENT AND SUGGESTED SOLUTIONS

JAWAHAR N. GHIA

During the past 25 years there has been a surge of interest in setting up pain clinics where patients with complex chronic pain can be examined and assessed with a promise of treatment. Because one person cannot encompass all the techniques and procedures that can be applied to the problem, such a clinic should be interdisciplinary and provide a well-integrated approach to pain problems. The effectiveness of interdisciplinary pain clinics and pain centers in management of patients with chronic, intractable pain is now well documented.[1–6] The most promising approaches to treatment have come out of interdisciplinary pain centers such as the one established at the University of North Carolina (UNC), whose evolution, organization, and function have been previously addressed.[7–9]

In 1972 we reported some problems that jeopardize the development and continued existence of pain centers.[10] One purpose of this chapter is to identify problems inherent in organizing a pain center and to provide a critical appraisal of problems affecting the field of pain management in general and those who manage it. A second purpose is to introduce caution, not pessimism, by focusing on the consequences of each problem as they relate to the future development of pain centers and to discuss some ways to approach the problems. Some practical guidelines for pain evaluation and treatment are offered along the way. Within such a framework, the task of treating chronic pain can be made more easily manageable for any newly formed group.

TERMINOLOGY: ITS INFLUENCE ON PAIN APPRAISAL AND MANAGEMENT

The pain experience

In the last 30 years significant advancement has been made in the understanding and management of pain. However, pain is one of the most subjective complex human experiences, one whose complete understanding is elusive. The term *pain* is used here to refer to "an unpleasant sensory and emotional experience typically associated with actual or potential tissue damage or described in terms of such damage."[11]

There is no general agreement among the experts in the field about the nature of the pain experience, classification of chronic pain states, underlying etiologies, pain mechanisms, or ways to manage pain. However, interest in the management of pain patients has increased significantly. Even though the role of tissue injury as a generator of pain is still emphasized in various neurophysiologic laboratories, pain in the absence of appropriate organic damage is very common in actual medical practice. The nature of psychological, social, ethnocultural, cognitive, environmental, and biochemical stimuli is not fully understood; mechanisms by which these stimuli cause pain are unknown. Attempts to understand all the known aspects of personhood and their relationship to illness and suffering present problems of phenomenal complexity and magnitude.

"Chronic" pain: an ambiguous generalization

Description of pain as acute or chronic has its share of problems. Pain associated with an acute disease, traumatic injury, or inflammation is termed *acute pain*, whereas chronic pain is arbitrarily defined as that which lasts longer than six months or beyond the normal course of the disease or injury.[12–13] Acute pain is generally characterized by a "well-defined temporal pattern of pain onset, subjective and objective physical signs, and hyperactivity of the autonomic nervous system."[14] Acute pain is largely self-limiting or, if accurately diagnosed early and properly managed, does not constitute a serious, long-term problem.

To patients, all pain is unpleasant whether acute or chronic, and relief of subjective symptoms is more meaningful than judgments by clinicians and researchers. The term *chronic* has many meanings. Often patients associate the word with hopeless, incurable conditions, and interpretation of this term varies widely even among pain managers. In the absence of data on the normal healing time for disease processes that cause pain, the term *chronic pain* does not suggest a specific duration to pain physicians.

The term *chronic* can be confusing when it is used to describe etiology or pain mechanism. To some physicians it may mean that the pain is persistent and ongoing with no clearcut, underlying etiology; psychological problems are perceived as the basis of pain that resists conventional medical and surgical treatments. To other physicians, chronic pain appears due to a heterogeneous group of syndromes with diverse etiologies.

Chronic pain can be represented in a broad spectrum (figure 6–1). Representa-

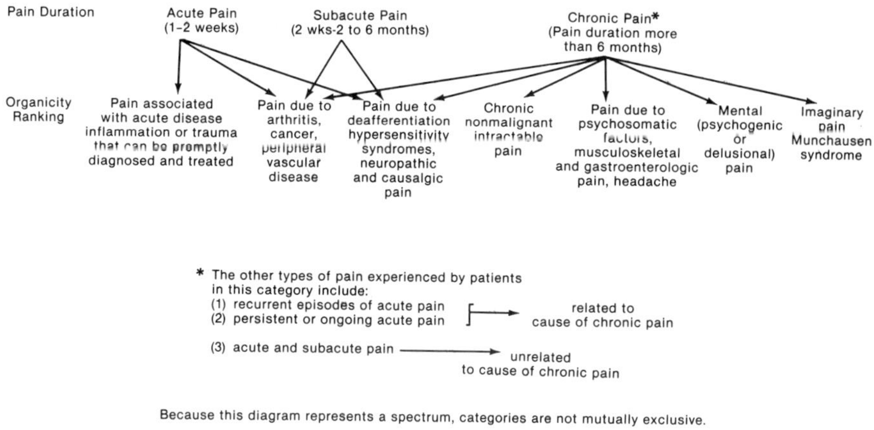

Figure 6-1. Spectrum of pain according to pain duration and organicity

tive of the spectrum are pain due to malingering pain from hallucinations secondary to possible biochemical derangement as in schizophrenia, pain from chronic degenerative disease and/or persistent neurologic conditions associated with arthritis, pain from complex interaction between tissue injury and psychopathology as in chronic nonmalignant intractable pain syndrome, and obvious tissue injury associated with posttraumatic states and cancer. To experienced clinicians dedicated to managing pain, chronic pain, which encompasses heterogeneous conditions with unknown etiologies, diverse pain mechanisms, and unknown cures, is not a single entity. Without further definition of subcategories, the terms *acute* and *chronic pain* do not recommend specific therapeutic strategies. Treatments for muscle spasm, abscess, appendicitis, or postoperative pain vary just as widely as treatments for chronic pain secondary to schizophrenia, chronic intractable nonmalignant pain, or cancer. Treating all pain the same way regardless of etiology is not logical, nor will it reliably result in successful pain control.

The use of the term *chronic pain* is a double-edged sword. Its advantages are (1) it has separated acute pain from chronic pain (2) it has exposed the enormous social and economic burden of the chronic sufferer and finally, (3) it has generated curiosity and enthusiasm in health professionals. Its disadvantages are (1) the term could have three different meanings when interpreted in literary, medical, and pain clinic settings by patients, physicians, and pain managers, respectively; (2) it reduces understanding of a complex phenomenon to a deceptively simple level, overshadowing the need for clinicians to study the pathophysiology of each chronic pain syndrome and to define more useful pain mechanisms whose evaluation is difficult and time consuming; and (3) it leads most clinicians to believe that all chronic pain is identical and responds to identical treatment modalities.

Despite these disadvantages the terms *acute* and *chronic* are widely accepted by clinicians worldwide in an uncritical way. Every article on pain emphasizes the need to understand differences between acute and chronic pain. Some pain managers describe differences between acute and chronic pain in brochures distributed to their patients prior to initial pain clinic visits. These labels of acute and chronic pain deliver a simple message: that the origin, treatment, and natural history of acute and chronic pain are entirely different and that a single treatment modality for all pain regardless of its etiology is not logical—a fundamental and intuitive statement.

Perhaps the overemphasis of acute and chronic pain labels without specific meanings may be the modern expression of the truth that we do not know enough about the essential nature of pain. Or, perhaps it merely represents extension of the familiar stance assumed by physicians in earlier days who believed in the specificity theory of pain and described pain using old notions such as "real or imaginary," or "organic and functional," and "peripheral and central." Use of the word *chronic*, however, is considerably less offensive to patients than "imaginary" pain, with its implications of malingering, or "functional" pain, with a psychogenic element. If mechanisms of pain can be understood, the clinical differences between the acute and chronic pain will become less important.

Chronic pain redefined

It is convenient and helpful to others to use words that have an agreed-upon technical meaning. The term *chronic pain* needs to be redefined to prevent stereotyping patients who belong to this group. The term chronic pain presents the physician with a number of features distinguishing it from acute pain:

1. An extended duration, persisting for several months or longer beyond the normal course of the disease or injury (fully realizing limitations of norms for length based on clinical impressions).
2. An ill-defined pain mechanism.
3. Poor or no response to conventional pain management.
4. Associated change in normal behavior patterns.
5. A set of learned behaviors that appear to have been shaped by secondary gains in addition to nociceptive input and to contribute to suffering. Suffering behaviors may provide important solutions to lifelong problems of dependency, inadequacy, and insecurity. In many instances the patients resist attempts to cure their suffering, which may fulfill some psychological need.
6. Many subgroups with possibly physical, behavioral, and psychological heterogenity among the chronic pain population.
7. Partial responsiveness to well-integrated interdisciplinary pain clinic treatment strategies that match physical, medical, biological, and psychological styles and needs.

The classification of pain syndromes

Although there are many classifications of organic pain syndromes in the literature, a standardized and clinically useful classification of pain disorders commonly

Talbe 6–1. Clinical classification of pain disorders

Congenital Absence of Pain

I. Congenital indifference to pain

II. Congenital insensitivity to pain with anhydrosis

III. Familial central autonomic dysfunction
Subtotal or total absence of unmyelinated fibers in the peripheral somatic and autonomic nervous systems

IV. Certain hereditary or acquired neuropathies
Hyperlastic myelinopathy and hereditary sensory radicular neuropathy

Acute Pain

I. Pain associated with injury
Broken bones or muscle strains/sprains
Severe posttraumatic pain
Burn pain, pains from cuts, bruises and electrical shock

II. Acute inflammatory disease
Abscess
Appendicitis
Cholecystitis
Acute toothache
Acute salpingo-oophoritis

III. Medical diagnostic/therapeutic procedures
Bone marrow biopsy
Surgery (postoperative pain)
Tooth extraction

IV. Visceral disease
Acute myocardial infarction
Renal colic

V. Acute abdominal pain in general medical conditions
Diabetes mellitus
Tabes dorsalis
Sickle cell anemia
Acute intermittent porphyria
Opiate withdrawal
Lead poisoning

VI. Pain of multiple etiologies
Acute headache

VII. Acute pain associated with incurable disease
Acute cancer pain associated with tumors and cancer therapy

VIII. Pain experimentally induced in a laboratory
Tourniquet pain
Electrical shock
Compression of the Achilles tendon

IX. Physiologic episodes of acute pain
Joint pain, tenesmus
Labor pain
Pain of daily living not associated with disease or injury
Earache, muscle spasm
Joggers' pain

Chronic Pain

Group I. Chronic pain due to progressively incurable and/or terminal diseases
1. Cancer pain due to tumor progression and chemotherapy

Group II. Chronic pain due to unsucessful traditional management of the classic pain syndromes (and conditions that mimic them) of various etiologies e.g.; congenital, inflammatory, posttraumatic, degenerative, neurologic, vascular, metabolic, postsurgical, or any combination of these

1. Torticollis
2. Chronic pancreatitis, chronic pelvic inflammatory disease, posterior parametritis
3. Myofascial pain dysfunction syndromes
4. Arthritis of spine and joints (osteoarthritis, rheumatoid arthritis)
5. Whiplash injuries
6. Posttraumatic neuropathy
7. Coccydynia
8. Posttraumatic headache
9. Shoulder-hand syndrome
10. Causalgia
11. Reflex sympathetic dystrophy
12. Herniated lumbar disc
13. Tabes dorsalis (a degenerative condition associated with untreated syphilis)
14. Temporomandibular joint syndrome
15. Nerve compression syndromes (carpal tunnel syndrome, meralgia paraesthetica, ilioinguinal pain syndrome)
16. Deafferentation syndromes, e.g. phantom limb pain, postherpetic neuralgia, brachial plexus avulsion, and spinal cord injury
17. Multiple sclerosis
18. Demyelinating disease such as disseminated sclerosis
19. Central pain such as tic douloureux (trigeminal neuralgia)
20. Pain associated with nerve root damage and arachnoiditis
21. Ischemic pain associated with peripheral vascular disease, e.g. thromboangiitis obliterans or arteriosclerosis obliterans
22. Raynaud's disease
23. Chronic abdominal pain due to gastric ulcer, duodenal ulcer, and irritable bowel syndrome
24. Chest pain, e.g., pleuritic pain, cardiac pain, angina pectoris
25. Mittelschmerz, premenstrual tension, endometriosis
26. Gout
27. Diabetic peripheral neuropathy
28. Osteoporosis
29. Paget's disease
30. Hemophilia
31. Dysmenorrhea
32. Painful scars, e.g., postmastectomy pain, painful postoperative scars, pain in burn scars
33. Postoperative pain following cholecystectomy (postcholecystectomy syndrome), nephroureterolithotomy

Group III. Chronic nonmalignant intractable pain due to complex multifactorial pathogenesis

1. Back pain
2. Orofacial pain
3. Headache
4. Visceral pain (abdominal and thoracic pain)
5. Pelvic and perineal pain
6. Cervical and/or shoulder pain

Group IV. Chronic pain associated with psychopathology involving behavioral, psychological, and psychiatric disorders and no evidence of tissue injury directly contributing to pain (psychogenic pain)

1. Chronic pain due to malingering, Munchausen syndrome
2. Affective disorders such as depression
3. Somatization disorders such as hypochondriasis
4. Conversion reactions (pain of hysterical origin)
5. Schizophrenia, organic psychoses, dementias (pain of delusional origin)
6. Personality disorders such as the dependent personality, the hysterical personality, and the pain-prone personality

7. Musculoskeletal pains (muscle-tension headache, backache, bodyache) due to psychoneurotic anxiety reaction
8. Adjustment disorders
9. Substance-use (abuse) disorders
10. Compensation neurosis
11. Chronic pain due to religious beliefs
12. Chronic pain as a symptom of unresolved grief
13. Chronic pain from stress due to severe chronic physical problems with repeated medical and surgical interventions
14. Chronic pain in patients with emotional and psychological disturbances due to iatrogenic factors

---

encountered in a university hospital is lacking. A classification of pain disorders is presented here (table 6–1) in which pain disorders are classified by the presence or absence of pain, by chronology (i.e., acute versus chronic), and according to pain syndromes (e.g., causalgia, angina pectoris, and the like). Interdisciplinary pain centers must make every effort to study a broad range of disorders beginning from the congenital absence of pain to the full spectrum of acute and chronic pain.

Congenital indifference to pain

Congenital indifference to pain is a well-recognized entity in which neuropathological examination of verified cases has failed to reveal any abnormality. It is possible to distinguish this syndrome from another condition, congenital insensitivity to pain with anhydrosis, in which the tract of Lissauer and small dorsal root ganglion neurones are absent.[15]

Acute pain

Acute pain is most commonly caused by the application of some harmful agent. This may be a knife, excessive pressure, or the extremes of heat and cold. Chemicals too may cause pain following their injection or local release in conditions of tissue damage (i.e., burns, peritonitis, ischemia). Postoperative pain, toothache, labor pain, and pain associated with certain therapies are examples of acute pain. Some, but not all, tumors are painful. Perhaps the amount of pain associated with some tumors is related to their rapid expansion into hard tissues, causing compression of nerve fibers, a local richness of nociceptive fibers, or liberation of more chemical pain mediators in some tissues than in others. Regrettably, we do not have an adequate electrophysiological explanation of the pain generated by amputation neuromata or nerve entrapment.

Acute pain may be well localized or poorly localized depending on the tissue of origin. Referred pain due to visceral disease has a distribution that follows known dermatomes, but that of deep somatic stimulation does not. That the location of the referred pain and associated phenomena are relatively constant and predictable suggests that referred pain also follows fixed anatomic pathways that are unknown at the present time. Thus, contrary to popular belief, acute pain may not always be associated with clearcut etiologies, known pain mechanisms, and well-defined pathways.

Chronic pain

Patients with chronic pain who visit the pain clinic can be divided into four groups: *group I*: those with a known cause of pain for which no effective treatment has been discovered (e.g., cancer, arthritis); *group II*: those with clear diagnoses although traditional treatment has failed to produce relief (e.g., unsuccessfully treated patients with the classic pain syndromes and conditions that mimic them); *group III*: those whose causes of pain are not fully known, for whom only the interdisciplinary approach has partially controlled the pain (e.g., chronic, nonmalignant intractable pain); or *group IV*: those whose cause of pain has not been determined (psychogenic pain). It is important to understand that these groups are not mutually exclusive. For example, a patient with a lifelong history of neck pain due to myofascial pain dysfunction syndrome may develop pain in the chest due to lung cancer and metastasis. Also, in many situations associated phyical disorders, concurrent psychopathology and/or interactions with premorbid personality are very common, thus complicating the overall picture. For example, a patient with carcinoma of the lung develops chest pain that cannot be shown to be due to metastasis but responds to treatment of depression.

How the neglected acute pain becomes chronic

Mismanagement of pain is extremely common in all groups. The following discussion uses patients in group II (table 6–1) as an example because they represent a group that is thought to have "acute" pain due to "clearcut" etiologies by traditional physicians. Lumbar strain, whiplash, and lumbar disc disease are all supposed to have reversible pathophysiology that causes pain and disability, and they have enjoyed acceptance as disease entities even though not understood. Although some patients in this group do well with appropriate traditional pain management, many fail to get prolonged relief because our poor understanding of pain mechanisms causes mismanagement. Examples of mismanagement include (1) inappropriate diagnosis due to failure to distinguish between classic pain syndromes and conditions that mimic them, (2) failure to establish an early definitive diagnosis before the condition becomes chronic, (3) incomplete diagnosis, (4) failure to evaluate the role of underlying pain mechanisms, and finally, (5) failure to appreciate the role of psychopathology. Further mismanagement of these patients includes (1) inadequate or inappropiate treatment (undertreatment, overtreatment, or lack of treatment), (2) wrong treatment, (3) failure to treat psychopathology, and (4) iatrogenic problems from mismanagement requiring further treatments.

Since there are no accurate statistics available on the differential effectiveness of traditional therapy in classic pain syndromes, traditional physicians continue to treat them as acute pain based on their limited successes. It can be truly stated that if acute pain were approached more astutely, there would be less chronic pain. Prevention of chronic syndromes appears to be the best way to manage acute pain patients. Traditional physicians should be encouraged to consult pain managers in the early phases of classic pain syndrome management because inadequately treated patients from group II may develop chronic intractable pain. Intractable pain has been defined as pain that has been present over a month and unremitting despite treatment. Patients with chronic nonmalignant intractable pain (group III), which is now a well-recognized entity, are most commonly seen in pain clinics.[18-20] (Chronic nonmalignant intractable pain is referred to as "chronic benign pain" by some investigators even though there is nothing benign about the chronic pain. Patients having chronic benign pain are described as having chronic pain syndrome, chronic benign intractable pain syndrome, or chronic disability syndrome.)

Conceptualization and management

A major problem in managing chronic pain is differing conceptualizations of the genesis of pain. The disease model assumes that symptoms or illness events are controlled by some underlying pathologic factor or antecedent stimulus[21-22] and frequently ignores the fact that behavior is partially governed by consequences in the environment. The learning model[23], however, assumes that the longer the patient has pain, the more important is the influence of psychologic factors on neurophysiologic mechanisms underlying pain behavior; illness that is composed primarily of behavior and chronicity is in need of behavior change. In this framework, symptoms are to the disease model as behavior is to the learning model.[21] The learning model view of patients with chronic intractable pain seems more rational. However, behavioral approaches have considerable limitations[24], and their application as primary therapy for all patients with chronic pain is open to question.

Indeed, in many, and perhaps the majority, of pain patients seen in private practice, operant mechanisms cannot be identified. Many factors contribute to the pathogenesis of chronic pain, which can appear to become a uniform syndrome after a certain length of time, often resembling depression, regardless of the nature and amount of disease initially involved. In actuality, physical, psychological, and behavioral characteristics of various patients in this group are not so homogeneous as previously thought.[25-26] For these reasons, treatment modalities adopted by pain programs that adhere to a particular conceptualization of this syndrome are not likely to be uniformly successful. For example, many clinics claim to be interdisciplinary but prescribe almost exclusively operant conditioning treatment. They report their treatment results by assessing factors that most readily lend themselves to such measurement.

The study of pain syndromes, pain mechanisms, and pain conduction pathways

Many busy pain clinicians, out of necessity, take the empiric approach of easing pain and do not investigate basic mechanics. This is best exemplified by the prevailing attitude of some physicians that if a low-morbidity, low-cost therapy works well enough, it matters little whether it does so by physiologic or emotional mechanisms.[27] Although methods of testing pain mechanisms in the normal pain-free man[28] and in persons complaining of pain[29] have been described, there is no uniform, sensitive, and reliable method available to investigate pain mechanisms in a clinical setting. Since there is no general agreement among physicians about the magnitude of suffering from poorly defined pain syndromes, no serious attempts are made to study pain mechanisms.

Tradition has also been a serious deterrent to the study of pain mechanisms not associated with tissue damage. After all, most health professionals serving in the pain clinic probably have not received formal training in pain and its control. Because their earlier training emphasized that every pain originates from a specific physical cause, these physicians spend an inordinate amount of time and effort establishing a link between tissue damage and pain complaint. At the same time they tend to underutilize or neglect other medical and psychologic resources to arrive at a diagnosis. Most diagnostic errors result from clinicians' heavy dependence on clinical impressions and interpretations of radiologic and laboratory data. We feel that certain prerequisites and systematic evaluation are necessary to establish a definitive diagnosis in patients with complex chronic pain problems before any treatment can be initiated (table 6–2). Shortcuts in these steps can lead to missed diagnosis and failed treatment.

In the diagnostic process, nerve blocks can be very useful to provide information on the mechanism and pathways of the patient's pain and to help predict the effects of neurosurgery or neurolytic blocks.[30–32] Unfortunately, the diagnostic nerve block techniques have not been utilized to their full potential in the management of chronic pain patients.

Table 6–2. Basic requirements of interdisciplinary evaluation to establish a definitive pain diagnosis

Prerequisites

1. Knowledge of pathophysiology of various chronic pain syndromes.
2. Knowledge of the neurological and psychological mechanisms of pain.
3. Sustained interest and dedication in study of pain.
4. Experience in managing pain problems, preferably in a multidisciplinary pain clinic setting.
5. A working knowledge in the fields of neurology, neurosurgery, anesthesiology, physical medicine, and psychiatry.

Individualized evaluation

1. Interpret history, physical examination, radiologic studies, and laboratory data to determine the cause of the pain; its site, intensity, and probable duration; and the nature of the disease causing pain.
2. Evaluate complicating psychopathology, premorbid personality, and complicating physical disorders.
3. Arrive at clinical (medical and psychiatric) diagnosis and differential diagnosis. Define etiologic factors and anatomic diagnosis.
4. Delineate pain mechanisms with the use of a differential nerve block technique, for examples sympathetic, somatic, central or psychogenic.
5. Establish a cause-and-effect relationship between the observed pathology and pain by blocking the appropriate pain pathways.[31]
6. Integrate above findings with the opinions of consultants to arrive at a definitive medical diagnosis.

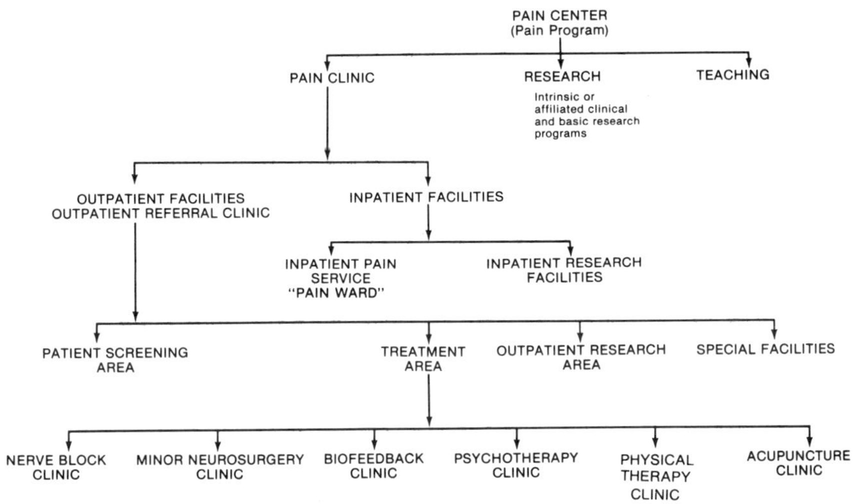

Figure 6-2. What is a pain center?

EVOLUTION OF A PAIN CENTER IN A MEDICAL CENTER

Distinction between a pain center and pain clinic

There is generally no agreement, even among experts, about the use of the terms *pain clinics* and *pain centers*. Larger organized facilities that have a broader scope than pain clinics are usually termed *pain centers* (figure 6–2). In addition to handling global management of referrals, they undertake teaching and research to study the full spectrum of the congenital absence of pain, acute pain, and chronic pain. Many pain "clinics" that cater primarily to private patients also call themselves pain "centers." Because private patients often associate the work "clinic" with charity or indigent outpatient units, sophisticated pain centers in the university setting often call themselves "pain programs." The term *pain clinic* is used loosely throughout the chapter to describe any facility that handles pain referrals for the purposes of diagnosis and/or treatment.

It is also important to understand the distinction between multidisciplinary and interdisciplinary. A multidisciplinary approach suggests that many specialists from different disciplines are treating the patient, but there is no indication that communication exists among specialists about their different goals. By our own definition, interdisciplinary suggests communication among disciplines with all specialists working toward common goals. We consider the most effective pain center an interdisciplinary one.

Growth of pain centers

Many innovative approaches, as well as more individualized combinations of modalities, have grown out of the interdisciplinary concept. A medical center is well equipped for teaching modern techniques to practicing physicians who eventually will become responsible for controlling patients' pain. Despite the many advantages of an interdisciplinary approach claimed by pain managers worldwide, comprehensive centers appear to have difficulty surviving while specialized pain clinics are thriving. The pain centers in the nation's teaching hospitals operate at a competitive disadvantage because of their dual role: (1) teaching and research and (2) providing care for all, including poor and indigent patients, many of whom are insurance risks or dropouts. A limited number of pain centers are doing well. Lack of stability and institutional support in the crucial developmental phase and heavy dependence on limited funding programs have discouraged other disciplines' participation in centers. Thus, single-specialty clinics minimize the potential of failure. These problems are not specific to any medical center. They reflect well-recognized incompatibilities between disciplines and the administrative structure of the typical center. There is also conflict with tradition since new programs may be viewed with great suspicion.

Along with limited progress in the development of responsible, comprehensive pain centers, unchecked growth in pain clinics has led to undesirable practices and abuse. Concerns shown by the pioneers in the field are as follows: (1) unreal expectations within the community based on the seductive promise of this modern scientific age that no one should ever have to suffer; (2) the exploitation of pain clinics as a means of insuring maximal financial gain for patients involved in workers' compensation or motor vehicle litigation; (3) media support for virtually any alternative to traditional Western medicine, from faith healing to acupuncture; (4) facilities run by physicians, other health professionals, or nonphysicians who may be unscrupulous or have had no training or experience in managing chronic pain patients; (5) abuse of these facilities by very reputable physicians who wish to broaden their personal images or their departments' images; and finally, (6) exploitation by patients who are looking for "new treatments" to cure their pain.

Starting a center

It is essential that the problems that militate against the establishment of pain centers be overcome if we are to consolidate the gains we have made in reducing the burden of chronic pain. There are no simple remedies. We must recognize that within the medical community and in hospital administration the study and treatment of chronic pain are separate entities. Many traditions in medicine must be overcome if an interdisciplinary program is to achieve acceptance and permanent financial support.

ADMINISTRATIVE IMPEDIMENTS IN A MEDICAL CENTER

The administrative impediments affecting the development of pain centers have been described elsewhere.[10] Fully salaried, most pain physicians are on both attending and housestaff levels and may not be cost-conscious when administering patient care. Whether patients pay their pain clinic bills is of little or no consequence to them. Their top priorities, and rightly so, are patient care, teaching, and learning. The relative novelty and unconventional programs of pain clinics has impeded support from hospital administrators and reimbursement from third-party carriers. This predicament is exacerbated by the expense of the interdisciplinary team approach. Governmental health programs aggravate matters by requiring supplemental reports and rarely reimbursing the full charge. All those factors complicate billing and collection. Funding from research grants and departmental contributions are usually inadequate and too uncertain to achieve necessary cost-effectiveness.

The visibility and growth of a pain center depend on a strong director. However, this position's effectiveness is frequently compromised by lack of support, unwillingness of hospital administrators to clearly define the director's position within the hospital hierarchy, or by the climate affecting the academic specialty the director represents.

The pain clinic's space and staffing needs are unique compared to other hospital clinics because the clinic tries to perform and integrate diverse functions in an interdisciplinary environment with only a few specialists interested in pain management. The public, other health professionals, and hospital administrators do not appreciate these needs and give them low priority. The price of satisfying these needs is often too high for the operation to break even.

The pain center director needs direct access to administrators of the involved institutions; the director must obtain consent from individual department heads to release their faculty for work in the pain center and to recognize their pain-related research in evaluation for promotions. A full-time director and adequate ancillary personnel can help assure that the center operates effectively and cooperatively. Given the realities of today's medicine, the administrative manager should be committed to planning and carrying out a cost center approach to financial management. The establishment of an autonomous, flexible trust fund with disbursement to participating faculty according to their level of clinical activity could strengthen the program.

MEDICAL TRADITION AND INTERDISCIPLINARY PROGRAMS

Professional development

Traditional departments and individuals within the medical center are often unsympathetic to new programs because they lack knowledge in the pain management field. They may be supspicious and resistant to change. In addition, many other factors reduce efficiency and deplete the physician's energy, possibly leading to professional burnout. Among these are (1) lack of interdisciplinary team support; (2) lack of commitment for personnel, space, and financial support from the dean of the clinic or the departments involved; (3) lack of financial support for attendance by outside consultants and specialists; (4) lack of coverage for sick leave, vacation, and absences; (5) absence of gratification due to failures of pain therapy; and (6) failure of colleagues and peers to recognize the value of working in the pain clinic. As each of these impediments is overcome, the physician's morale is proportionately improved.

Patient care

Philosophical differences between medical traditions and interdisciplinary programs also become apparent at various levels of patient care. This conflict may begin when a traditional physician refers a patient to the pain clinic for a specific procedure, a treatment that may be contraindicated according to pain managers who emphasize a holistic approach to the patient's pain problem. Pain managers must appease the referring physician and at the same time do their best for the patient. Also, this type of specific referral can deter pain managers from getting a second opinion from other consultants.

Different conceptions by pain consultants from different disciplines can result in heated discussions about complex issues that have no clearcut answers. For example, psychiatrists may believe that answers for chronic pain will not come from the field of neurophysiology. They view knowledge of pain receptors and encephalins as exciting discoveries but predict many years of development before they become useful for pain management. They feel that neurophysiological treatments will never substitute for experience, a personal approach, and treatment of the patient rather than the symptom. Patients frequently become victims when these conflicts result in utter chaos. Only when center personnel respect the offerings of their colleagues from other disciplines—rather than compete for dominance by their specialties, diagnosis, treatment recommendations, and progress assessment—can patients benefit from these diverse perspectives.

DAILY OPERATIONAL ACTIVITIES

Patterns of referral

The pain clinic frequently becomes a target of patient referral as a means to "dump" the patient rather than a place to get consultation. Once practicing physicians begin to appreciate the value of reliable and efficient service provided by the clinic, a change in the referral pattern may occur. Many "difficult patients" may be referred whose management may be a major problem for the practicing physician. These patients have multiple chronic problems across system lines, and they are frequent utilizers of health services. The pain clinic usually sees patients with "thick chart syndromes," that is, patients with voluminous records due to unresolved medical problems and/or chronic pain requiring frequent visits and/or hospitalizations. Once the pain clinic is well established, however, many patients with thin charts are also referred. Patients with thin charts are referred in the early stage of disease, before pain has become intractable or they have become addicted to narcotics. But patients frequently have not had an adequate workup before they are referred to the pain clinic.

Patient selection is the key factor in determining the type of program a pain treatment center will follow. For example, if no one on the staff is interested in pelvic pain, patients with this problem should not be selected. Since patients are referred by private physicians and third-party payers, every effort should be made to obtain and review patient records prior to admission for outpatient evaluation. The first level of the screening function can be the pain clinic secretary. By deft handling of patients over the telephone, the secretary can save patients a great deal of time by screening out those who obviously do not belong in the pain center. Rigid criteria for admission of patients with chronic pain must be followed, and postscreening options should be clearly defined.

Personnel and scheduling

In many clinics, the secretary functions as an appointment secretary, receptionist, telephone operator, social worker, and billing clerk. Unless the secretary is very efficient, chaos may result. The number of patients who can be seen is limited by the part-time nature of a pain center. Patients are frequently scheduled subject to the vagaries of physician availability, which is primarily based on their responsibilities to other specialties. Scheduling patients with chronic pain is extremely difficult because preadmission screening may not reveal the the problem's complexity. Elective patients may not show up promptly at their scheduled appointment time. New patients requiring urgent attention also complicate scheduling. When many patients require follow-up appointments, there is little room for new patients in the clinic schedule. As a result the unit becomes self-inhibiting, with the development of a waiting list. New patients must be graded by urgency, a difficult task without seeing the patient.

Patient billing

Clerical support depends on the size and hours of the clinic and must not be underestimated. Generally, a full-time secretary is needed for a clinic open five days a week. This secretary, who may be a personal secretary to the pain director and other physicians participating in the center, may not be able to fulfill the role of the billing clerk. A separate financial officer or billing clerk may be essential for efficient billing. Fiscal viability is difficult to achieve unless care is taken to adjust patient mix, to obtain some prepayments, and to obtain commitment for preferential charging for facilities. To reduce paperwork, a single, all-inclusive fee (exclusive of laboratory tests and surgical or other procedures) rather than individual, fee-for-service billing by pain clinic personnel may be most beneficial and, ultiimately, most cost-effective.

Composition and formation of the pain team and work biases

Personnel problems can be resolved by involving physicians from various specialties in pain management in an organized and systematic way. With time and effort, such involvement can be combined with the conventional practices of participating physicians' primary specialties. The idea that a specific team member or pain manager must manage each person's case is appealing to all patients. However, this may not always be feasible, especially when the patient's complex pain problems require simultaneous application of diverse modes of therapies.

One particularly delicate matter is the formation of the pain teams through which consultants work. Their composition and the contributions of each member should reflect the team's stance toward treatment, which depends on whether an anesthesiologist, psychologist, or physician from another discipline directs the team. Regardless of the various skills of staff members, they must work together.

It is obvious that personnel from different disciplines who are willing to coordinate their efforts benefit a pain team. Less obvious are the benefits to each member from serving on a pain team and their impact on other medical personnel. Data from studies and clinical experience suggest that students, house officers, and practitioners have inadequate understanding of chronic pain and its management[33–35] despite the remarkable advances in the study of pain[36–39] in the past 15 years. For example, many practicing anesthesiologists use nerve blocks as a major form of pain control for patients with chronic intractable pain of undeterminate cause (the most common type seen in the pain clinics), although there is no conclusive evidence that this practice is effective.[40–42] On the other hand, anesthesiologists may refrain from using diagnostic nerve block techniques, even though they have proven effective in delineating pain mechanisms.[31–32] The informed, rational, and safe use of nerve block techniques is promoted by the collaborative approach of the team. Team participation allows extension of the anesthesiologist's role beyond that of block technician. However, involvement in team efforts at pain management demands time and effort, more than some anesthesiologists are willing to spend unless they value their enhanced roles.

Utilization of consultants depends mainly on the type of patients and patient loading; however, "clustering" different pain consultants in one setting, as opposed to the more traditional model of specialist referral, is more cost-effective for some pain patients. For example, a patient with a long-standing history of postincisional pain due to possible neuroma accompanied by major psychopathology may be best managed by a pain team with both a neurosurgeon and a psychiatrist. Without a team approach, the patient would be "handed off" between the two specialists, who might not coordinate the patient's treatment.

Space (physical plant and design)

Pain clinics function from various locations. If the director is an anesthesiologist, the clinic may function close to the operating room. Indeed, the utility room, the equipment room, the recovery room, the holding area for the operating room, the anesthesia induction room, the room where a cast is changed prior to taking an orthopedic patient to the operating room, and the day-op surgery suite have all been used for the purpose. This is especially true in the early stages of a pain clinic's evolution and meets the needs of a limited patient load. As patient volume increases, the director may find it difficult to get a more organized facility unless the department chairperson or hospital administrator is convinced of the increased demand for clinic services. Appropriate documentation may be necessary. Many times the process of renegotiation involves a long-term assignment of temporary space, repeated disruptions of patients by changing offices, and dwindling enthusiasm of the clinic's leaders. Sharing space with other clinics can also be chaotic if not properly organized.

The designs of physical facilities are sometimes difficult to conceptualize because models may not be available for comparison. Types of facilities may vary from one center to another depending upon patient load, expertise of individual consultants, and the nature of a research program. Because of the diverse nature of services offered by the pain clinic, it is extremely difficult to maintain close proximity of the related fuctions of consultation, evaluation, treatment, and recovery. This may compromise effectiveness of the interdisciplinary approach because related rehabilitation services cannot work together to achieve optimal patient care.

Adequate facilities are vital in the treatment of chronic pain. Since patient morale varies from low to rock bottom and most patients have been treated before unsuccessfully, it is therefore unlikely that a 20 minute outpatient interview will solve complex problems. Pain clinics rarely have their own inpatient beds. An arrangement must be made to allow hospital admission for the following problems:

1. Surgical procedures for pain relief.
2. Major nerve block.
3. Use of continuous infusion techniques.
4. Interdisciplinary invasive workup.
5. Drug detoxification.
6. Complex psychiatric problems associated with chronic pain.
7. Initial stages of an extensive behavior modification and rehabilitation program.
8. Suicidal tendencies/depression.
9. Currently hospitalized patients who require pain therapy during their hospitalization.

Assessment of chronic pain problems

Need for a standard protocol for evaluation

Unfortunately, there are no standardized processes for the evaluation of chronic pain nor scientifically approved protocols for treatment. Many contributing factors, inherent in each patient's makeup, contribute to pain. Anxiety, depression, and socioeconomic factors superimposed on organic factors play important roles. The relative importance of these components must be assessed before a regimen is selected. Unfortunately, objective methods of assessment are hopelessly inadequate for comparing the results of assessment in a defined group of patients or between different groups of patients.

The measurement of clinical, pathologic pain has eluded accurate appraisal for many years.[43–44] Since there is no simple physiologic or biological marker for identifying whether someone has a chronic pain problem, the scientific study of pain is forced to approach pain as a subjective phenomenon. Nonetheless, subjective report of pain is vital for diagnosis, treatment, and theoretical understanding. It reflects the degree of suffering, which is important in clinical medicine; it increases our understanding of human behavior in the face of suffering; and it provides a means for evaluating analgesics.

Many investigators in the field of pain consider the lack of an objective measure to quantitate pain as the single biggest obstacle in "pain" evaluation. Although the need for such a method cannot be denied, strong emphasis on this issue is debatable. Most recent advances in understanding pain mechanisms, neuroanatomy, and neurophysiology have come about without such a system of "pain" evaluation. Clinicians do not use or need such a system when they manage acute pains with clearcut etiologies. For example, a surgeon does not use any sophisticated system to quantitate pain in the patient who has acute appendicitis before deciding to do an appendectomy! Postoperatively, the patient receives narcotics as needed and the verbal report of pain from the patient is considered trustworthy. On the other hand, the chronic pain patient whose symptom has resisted treatment and who continues to report pain is considered a less credible witness, and an objective measure of the distress is sought.

Although many approaches have been suggested to quantitate pain, no single approach has been found to be simple, practical, and uniformly successful. The biggest challenge is how to measure the consequences of environmental, cognitive, behavioral, biological, and emotional aspects of pain. An acute quest of some investigators to reduce these nonphysical factors to mathematical numbers has oversimplified the complex phenomenon of chronic pain. Physicians' insistence on measuring suffering by numbers can reinforce chronic pain behavior. Perhaps the anxiety of investigators who feel a need for such a system would decrease were pain mechanisms identified for many chronic pain syndromes.

Principles of pain evaluation

The two principles of pain evaluation should be (1) accurate physical diagnosis and (2) accurate and comprehensive psychiatric and psychosocial evaluation. Unfortunately these principles are violated repeatedly, and treatment before diagnosis is common in a majority of pain clinics.

Accurate physical diagnosis requires a thorough review of the patient's records; a detailed history including pain; medical/surgical, social, occupational, personal, and drug history; and a detailed, precise physical examination. Unfortunately, all standardized neurological examination protocols of the sensory nervous system lack the detail addressed by the neurophysiologist who is well trained in pain management. Pain physicians often spend too much time ordering tests of questionable value, taking x-rays, for medicolegal reasons and abusing electromyographic examination, and too little time on physical examination that could be more informative. Soft tissues are rarely exposed on x-rays, and comprehensive evaluation of the effects of injury on nerves, blood vessels, bones, muscles, ligaments, and psyche in posttraumatic cases is rarely done. Physical disorders such as myofascial pain dysfunction syndrome and reflex sympathetic dystrophy are commonly misdiagnosed. The diagnosis of psychiatric problems and depression are missed too often. Common use of vague labels such as "facet joint arthritis," "bursitis," and "psychogenic" often mislead patients. The rationale for placebo and nerve blocks to diagnose pain is poorly understood by many pain physicians. The results of the nerve blocks are frequently not explained to patients. Poor evaluation may result in the patient's failure to cooperate.

Psychological evaluation

Although the importance of psychological evaluation is well recognized by most pain clinics, there is no simple standardized method of psychiatric and psychological evaluation to study patients suffering from chronic pain. Nonetheless, recognition of behavioral and psychological problems allows for early treatment of chronic pain and may avoid unnecessary surgery and narcotic abuse.

A properly done psychological and/or psychiatric evaluation is always useful for diagnosis; however, the nature and extent of this evaluation varies according to the patient. Contacts with psychologists, psychiatrists, and mental health professionals not trained in chronic pain management are not very useful. Evaluation in a pain clinic setting may range from informal assessment of psychopathology by a pain manager to more formal measurement techniques employing screening inventories that include pain self-report, psychological assessment, and psychiatric interview.

When the pain manager suspects a strong psychological component, computer-administered rating scales may be useful screening tools to identify patients at risk for significant psychiatric morbidity. Rapid assessments of depression and anxiety identify those at risk for significant morbidity. Such assessments by microcomputer have been demonstrated by Hanks et al.[45] This test battery can be followed by a clinical interview, which is usually the initial contact between the patient and the psychologist in the interdisciplinary pain clinic setting. If the psychological report supports the suspicion of a psychophysiologic reaction, conversion reaction, or functional overlay, the pain manager can get a psychiatrist's opinion or initiate treatment.

Psychiatric referral may not always be necessary; in fact, the patient may refuse it with indignation. Chronic pain patients who loathe seeing a psychiatrist usually place themselves in a population with distinct clinical features. To obtain cooperation from this group, the pain manager must emphasize the necessity for the psychiatric/psychological evaluation as part of the holistic evaluation at the pain clinic. How the patient is informed of the diagnosis of psychogenic pain and how a referral to a mental health professional is made are very important.[46] In explaining that a referral to a mental health professional is indicated, it may be useful to suggest to the patient that emotions and induced stresses often affect bodily functions and vice versa, as for example, tension headaches, ulcers, and asthma. It should be acknowledged that the pain the patient sufffers is indeed being experienced and is not faked or caused by being "crazy" even if no physical cause is demonstrable. It may be helpful to suggest that by discussing ones life problems, one may relieve tensions that intensify or produce pain. It should be emphasized that the referring physician will continue to see, and will not abandon, the patient.

Assessment of treatment

Despite current progress in managing patients with chronic pain syndromes, therapeutic modalities that yield predictable results have not been developed. When the cause of intractable pain is unknown, symptomatic relief of pain and patient comfort become the clinical objectives. Regrettably, even these objectives are not always attainable.[4] Given multifactorial pathogenesis, it is not surprising that a single treatment method or treatment by only one medical specialist does not usually bring success. General principles of interdisciplinary management likely to be effective are provided in table 6–3. The wide range of treatment modalities employed requires close coordination by the interdisciplinary team so that the patient receives a consistent and holistic approach. Coordinated treatment also

Table 6–3. General therapeutic considerations in pain management

1. Establish a definitive diagnosis early in the disease and determine intervention on the basis of problem identification.
2. Treat all patients with chronic pain regardless of what started the pain and whether the process is still operative.
3. Carefully evaluate medical, social, and psychologic issues and treat them with goals rooted in the rehabilitation of the affected person.
4. Individualize therapy in conjunction with an eclectic approach to remove the limitation imposed by a select method of intervention such as operant conditioning or nerve blocks.
5. Create a trustful positive doctor-patient relationship by showing interest in the patient's pain problem and by carefully listening to his or her needs.
6. Do not get into a dialogue of "organic versus psychologic" causes with the patient.
7. Use a variety of treatment methods in combination rather than a single modality.
8. Educate patients about the multidimensional views of pain, the role of learning factors in pain behaviors, the ways to change pain behaviors, the reduction in the drug or alcohol dependence, the teaching of various coping skills, as well as goal setting and increased activity.
9. Educate patients to assume a more active role in managing their problems and establish a cooperative relationship.
10. Avoid invasive diagnostic and therapeutic procedures whenever possible.
11. Do not focus so much on "pain" or interruption of the pain pathways.
12. Use physiotherapy whenever possible. Apart from the specific benefits it imparts, physiotherapy has the effect of acknowledging in a tangible way the validity of patients' somatic pain statements, and therefore, their legitimate entitlement to the sick role.
13. Avoid polypharmacy.
14. Establish regular outpatient visits not contingent on the symptom.
15. Continue support despite failure of therapies.
16. Involve the family as a part of the team and treat them as an integral part of the treatment plan.
17. Use programmed exercises actively and passively to improve posture, flexibility, endurance, and strengh. Gradually translate the development of endurance into the resumption of vocational activities.
18. Convert the illness role of the patient to a well or health role and replace feelings of hopelessness and helpessness with positive feelings and hope for the future.
19. Reinforce the slighest improvement from the therapy, and as the functional level improves, develop new social skills unrelated to pain and disability.
20. Provide adequate long-term follow-up to maintain the gains.

helps the patient integrate skills and insights gained from specific disciplines.

Most pain clinics do not emphasize the importance of simple, cognitive approaches for pain control as much as physical, psychological, and behavioral approaches. The cognitive functions of knowledge, judgment, concentration, and the ability to think are useful tools in control of pain. Egbert, Battit, and Welch[47] showed that patients who had been prepared intellectually and psychologically, and who had good doctor-patient rapport, required significantly less analgesia and could be discharged from the hospital earlier than those who had not been prepared. Through suggestion, diversion, or knowledge, patients' awareness and ability to think can be used to alter favorably their perceptual pain response to noxious stimuli.[48]

Intriguing about the cognitive approach is that most patients can exert a certain amount of voluntary control to reduce the intensity of pain perception. Physicians can enhance this control by proper patient education and simple diversion tactics. Accurate patient education is a simple approach, one that is most effective. When applied as a single modality to increase patients' knowledge of the pain condition and to promote their adaptation behaviors, patient education may decrease pain and maintain function. For example, asking the patient to tolerate pain because nothing else can be done about it can sometimes reduce pain and suffering. Skills needed to avoid drug abuse, such as being assertive, clarifying values, making decisions, saying "no" to alcohol and other drugs, and overcoming need or peer pressure, can be taught. Also, it is amazing how little patients know about their bodies and the effect of drugs on their bodies and minds. Despite the apparent importance of patient education to chronic pain patients' care, few studies have evaluated the impact of education programs on patients' knowledge of chronic pain and behavior changes.[49–50]

Evaluation of the effectiveness of the interdisciplinary approach

The history and success of pain centers since their first development by Bonica are evident in the 1981 overview of interdisciplinary pain centers published by the National Institutes of Health.[51] Despite rapid growth in the number of pain clinics worldwide, there have been comparatively few reported studies of clinic effectiveness. The problems with studies that assess pain center success according to follow-up analysis include lack of comparison and control groups, use of self-report measures rather than more objective methods of assessing outcome, use of outcome measures with questionable validity and reliability, failure to use standardized instruments, lack of corroboration of self-reports, inadequate sample size, and dependence on the mailed questionnaire.[52] Despite the overall similarity of most clinic programs, it is still difficult to safely generalize about folow-up results because of methodological difficulties.

Despite considerable variations in their emphases and approaches, a majority of clinics report a high rate of success as judged by improvement in their patients' condition at discharge. A great majority of clinics directed by anesthesiologists and/or surgeons who do not recognize the importance of the psychological aspects of pain tend to be concerned largely with anesthetic and surgical methods of pain relief. For example, many anesthesiologists claim a high rate of success following the treatment of herpes zoster wth early nerve blocks even though this outcome is supported by only a few publications and lacks statistical verification.[53,54] On the other hand, many newly evolved inpatient units that concentrate on modifying pain-related behaviors as part of a multimodal approach claim and document a success rate of more than 70 percent initially and equally good results on follow-up.[55–58] Since many of these programs are predominantly behavioral in orientation, the data also support the hypothesis that learning factors are responsible for a significant portion of the chronic disability due to pain. Unfortunately, these studies rarely define the pain diagnoses of patients or the role of physical factors and their interactions with behavior. They rarely address pain mechanisms and common pathways through which behavioral strategies mediate pain relief.

Outcome criteria used to evaluate success of interdisciplinary pain management have not been standardized. Some investigators feel that the success of pain programs can probably be accurately assessed only by objective measures because of the tendency to underreport well-behavior.[59] Success rates therefore cannot serve as an accurate index of the effectiveness of therapeutic intervention. A simple and practical index, however, is to use subjective criteria with a rational approach.

Patients with chronic pain tend to manipulate subjective criteria because they fear losing secondary gains.[59] Patients may not exhibit well-behavior if they do not see the program as a supportive environment in which staff involvement and concern for their well-being compensate for the secondary gains they lose by getting well. It is important to spend time with patients, show interest in their problems, discuss the source of difficulty and expectations for the future, and help to solve socioeconomic and psychological problems. Patients who perceive the system as helpful and trust ongoing relationships with team members may be less fearful of revealing feelings or developing well-behavior.

Most pain clinics state their goals as the comprehensive conceptualization of the pain syndrome and rehabilitation of the chronic pain patient, yet most studies attempt to measure outcome in terms of the following: (1) reduction of pain; (2) reduction of medication intake; (3) improvement in "uptime" hours (hours spent out of bed) of increased activity level; and (4) the restoration of the occupational role. These narrow and constricted measures of improvement, although critical, do not assess the broad variety of patient roles that may demonstrate rehabilitation. Furthermore, patients do not understand these variables and often do not reveal progress indicators such as medications they are taking for fear they will be negatively evaluated and terminated. A clinic that relies upon a mailed questionnaire using these criteria collects data that depend upon the memory of the patients about events which took place at varying lengths of time before the questionnaire was completed.

The goals of the interdisciplinary pain center at the University of North Carolina Comprehensive Pain Program have been previously described[8] and are:

Table 6–4. Goals of interdisciplinary pain program

Pain management

1. To manage pain based on the cure, eradication, or control of the condition causing it. To offer interdisciplinary pain consultation and practical innovative approaches to frustrating pain problems for the physician or dentist.
2. To incorporate patient and family education in the management of chronic pain and improve family functioning.
3. To recognize the inherent dangers of iatrogenesis when diagnosis and management are obscure and to address this matter educationally with patients and health professionals.
4. To decrease the cost of medical care for chronic pain by reducing future patient dependence on the health care system.
5. To offer assistance with comprehensive assessment, functional impairment, and medical and social planning to all other interested parties such as insurance companies and lawyers.

Research

1. To conduct research in the medical, behavioral, surgical, dental, and anatomical aspects of various pain disorders, including congenital absence of pain, acute pain, and chronic pain.

Teaching

1. To offer educational opportunities for community physicians, and graduate and postgraduate students in medicine, dentistry and allied health fields.

Program quality assurance

1. To assess the effectiveness and efficiency of current treatment programs.

Table 6–5. Detailed description of interdisciplinary pain management goal and criteria used for pain management follow-up

A. *Aims*

1. Establishing a definitive diagnosis and program in an authoritative manner based on in-depth examination of physical, behavioral, social, and vocational factors contributing to the patient's symptomatology.
2. Developing an integrated treatment plan to relieve pain based on the cure, eradication, or control of the condition and to control pain behavior through medical, behavioral, and psychological techniques.
3. Relieving drug dependence by counseling and detoxification.
4. Advising the patient against unnecessary surgical procedures.
5. Educating the patient with regard to the anatomy, physiology, pharmacology, and psychiatry of his or her painful state and associated conditions.

Outcome measures

Decreasing pain and pain-related behaviors

Subjective criteria

1. Decrease in pain level (reduction in pain).
2. Decrease in verbalization of complaints and/or nonverbal pain behavior such as wincing, moaning, overcautious movement.
3. Reducation of disabilities brought on by pain.

Objective criteria

1. Change in attitude toward pain, for example acceptance of the need to live with pain.
2. Decrease in pain estimate or pain rating.
3. Decrease in number of hospitalizations.
4. Decrease in intake of pain-related and mood-enhancing medications and motivation to remain off medication.
5. Stopping abuse of medical therapies, quackeries, alcohol, coffee, tea, tobacco, cigarettes.
6. Decrease in use of unnecessary mutilative procedures for pain relief.

B. *Aims*

1. Restoring the patient's mood, emotional well-being, and psychological functioning to normal levels.
2. Resolving anxiety, depression, insomnia, constipation, obesity, inactivity, and other pain-related problems.
3. Improving community support systems.
4. Motivating the patient to get better.

Outcome measures

Increase in the self-management of subjective distress

Subjective criteria

1. Improvement in mood.
2. Decrease in fear, anxiety, depression, anger, frustration.
3. Improvement in outlook for life in general.
4. Improvement in self-esteem.
5. Improvement in sleep.
6. Able to cope efficiently with problems of daily living.
7. Enjoying life despite verbalization of pain.
8. Increased assertiveness.

Objective criteria

1. Improvement noted on psychological tests such as Zung Depression Inventory and psychiatric evaluation.
2. Reports of increased assumption of more responsibilities.
3. Good understanding of comprehensive nature of program and frequent application of self-initiation and self-reliance.
4. Comprehension of pain/anxiety relationship.

C. *Aims*

1. Restoring and improving the patient's level of functioning, that is, physical, social, familial, and the like.

Outcome measures

Increasing physical and social activity

Subjective criteria

1. Increase in social and work activities.
2. Increase in household activities, yard work, and shopping.
3. Carrying out programmed exercises.
4. Active educational and recreational pursuits.
5. Improvement in interpersonal relationships.
6. Return to satisfactory lifestyle.
7. Improvement in walking tolerance.
8. Improvement in family relationships.
9. Sexual adjustment and sexual relations.

Objective criteria

1. Improvement in "up time" hours (the time spent out of bed) or increase in activity level.
2. Weight reduction in obese patients.
3. Goniometry, to show improvement in joint movements.
4. Measures of physical functioning: (1) knee-to-chest, (2) average ability for active straight leg raise, (3) reaching for toes, and (4) overall exercise performance.
5. Reports of increase in recreational activities from spouse, friends, or relatives.
6. Achievement of other nonvocational goals in life.
7. Achievement of strength and functional physical performance.

D. *Aims*

1. Restoration of the occupational role.
2. Providing access to occupational rehabilitation.
3. Resetting goals so that they are realistic.
4. Assisting the patient in resolution of financial problems.

Outcome measures

Increasing vocational activity.

Subject criteria

1. Achievement of vocational goals.
2. Increase in tolerance for job-related activities.

Objective criteria

1. Settlement of compensation and litigation suits.
2. Levels of vocational restoration: Patient not yet able to consider vocational concepts due to physical disability and/or pain or status as employed (full-or part-time), in-training, running a household, or a student.
3. A review of work placement records.
4. Supervisor's assessment of type and quality of work and other work records.

E. *Aims*

1. Maintaining the gains made.
2. Regular follow-up visits to prevent patients from regressing.

Outcome measures

1. Adequate management of pain.
2. Patient accepting the concept of a useful and satisfying existence in spite of pain.
3. Increase in programmed activity and efficient self-care.
4. Reduction of pain medication.
5. Improvement in family relationships.

Subjective and objective criteria

A serial determination of global assessment of the above-mentioned criteria.

---

redefined in table 6–4. This chapter defines the outcome measures that are congruent with the stated pain management goal of the program (table 6–5). The main role of the pain program is to maximize the coping abilities of patients faced with intractable pain. We assess treatment outcome by measuring improvement in the patient's overall level of functioning, that is, social, occupational, familial, and the like. A global evaluation of the patient's self-report, a similar report from the patient's spouse, and a conference rating scale (figures 6–3 and 6–4) are completed at an initial interdisciplinary pain conference. The pain clinic consultants' ratings are used as baseline measures. The process is repeated immediately upon completion of an interdisciplinary treatment approach. Obtaining information in face-to-face interviews with patients before and after completion of the outpatient pain program avoids the problems inherent in self-report questionnaires. High scores on the subjective criteria used in each assessment reflect that, after treatment, the patient is living a life typical of someone his or her age and sex without interference from pain and without prescription medication.

The data are collected, stored, computerized, and evaluated by an impartial observer to interpret effectiveness of the interdisciplinary treatment. Pretreatment measures can be compared to posttreatment measures, and the same variables can be assessed on long-term follow-up by mailing questionnaires to the patients. If there is general agreement between pain programs for criteria of success, then comparative studies in the field are possible, provided each pain program will supply the following basic information:

Patient: ________ Spouse: ________ Clinician: ______ Date: ________

Circle the appropriate number

1. Pain relief

1 2 3 4 5 6 7 8 9 10
L O W M E D I U M H I G H

2. Relief of suffering

1 2 3 4 5 6 7 8 9 10
L O W M E D I U M H I G H

3. Confident that I do not need medicines or doctors to feel better

1 2 3 4 5 6 7 8 9 10
L O W M E D I U M H I G H

4. Lead normal stress-free life (good mood, enjoying life)

1 2 3 4 5 6 7 8 9 10
L O W M E D I U M H I G H

5. Able to cope effectively with problems of daily living

1 2 3 4 5 6 7 8 9 10
L O W M E D I U M H I G H

6. Willing to assume more responsiblilities

1 2 3 4 5 6 7 8 9 10
L O W M E D I U M H I G H

7. Get along better with others and socializing

1 2 3 4 5 6 7 8 9 10
L O W M E D I U M H I G H

8. Able to resume my physical functioning as before the pain began (daily activity, household work, sex)

1 2 3 4 5 6 7 8 9 10
L O W M E D I U M H I G H

9. Successful in achieving goals in my chosen role as homemaker, mother, father, breadwinner, or volunteer

1 2 3 4 5 6 7 8 9 10
L O W M E D I U M H I G H

10. Satisfied with my treatment

1 2 3 4 5 6 7 8 9 10
L O W M E D I U M H I G H

Figure 6–3. Patient's self-report of interdisciplinary treatment outcome

1. How many patients joined the program, how many left, how many completed it, reasons for leaving the program.
2. Program descriptions (e.g., medically oriented versus behaviorally oriented versus clinics that seek to integrate both approaches, inpatient versus outpatient).

Patient: ______________________ Clinician: ________ Date: ____________

Circle the appropriate number

1. Pain intensity

1 2 3 4 5 6 7 8 9 10
L O W M E D I U M H I G H

2. Pain suffering

1 2 3 4 5 6 7 8 9 10
L O W M E D I U M H I G H

3. Misuse of medication

1 2 3 4 5 6 7 8 9 10
L O W M E D I U M H I G H

4. Illness behavior reinforcement

1 2 3 4 5 6 7 8 9 10
L O W M E D I U M H I G H

5. Effect of pain on psychological function (anxiety, depression, hostility)

1 2 3 4 5 6 7 8 9 10
L O W M E D I U M H I G H

6. Overall stress

1 2 3 4 5 6 7 8 9 10
L O W M E D I U M H I G H

7. Pain interference with interpersonal relationships

1 2 3 4 5 6 7 8 9 10
L O W M E D I U M H I G H

8. Pain interference with physical activity (daily activity, household work, sex)

1 2 3 4 5 6 7 8 9 10
L O W M E D I U M H I G H

9. Pain interference with work

1 2 3 4 5 6 7 8 9 10
L O W M E D I U M H I G H

10. Realistic goals

1 2 3 4 5 6 7 8 9 10
L O W M E D I U M H I G H

Figure 6–4. Patient interdisicplinary conference rating scale

3. Average time spent per patient.
4. Cost of treatment.
5. Types of patients.
6. Types of problems.

Use of psychological predictors and admission criteria in selection of the best candidates for the pain management program

The value of psychological variables as predictors of health outcome depends on the adequacy of measures used. However, evaluation of currently used measuring instruments has produced mixed reviews. Some studies claim that these variables are effective in predicting success or failure.[60–61] Psychological diagnosis and psychometric information do not seem to be related to eventual success, a finding reported in earlier research.[62] A variety of indices of depression have been strongly associated with success or regression.

Many programs use psychological predictors as part of initial admission criteria to develop a quick and practical rating method to select good candidates for the interdisciplinary approach. However, before such a method becomes routinely accepted, it needs further validation and refinement through application to long-term follow-up of patients. If invalidated initial selection criteria are applied stringently (table 6–6) many deserving patients may be deprived of the interdisciplinary approach. If initial selection criteria are applied loosely, patients inappropriate to the program may be admitted, and high failure or drop out rates will result.

Some experienced programs, such as the one described by Swanson et al.[63], now recognize that some patients would exclude themselves if emphatically presented with the following treatment goals: (1) to live with pain, although no removal is assured; (2) to live with pain without pain-killing medications and sedatives; and (3) to work toward return to active physical functioning and employment. Patients with unrealistic expectations, delusional pain behavior, severe drug dependency, and extensive medicolegal complications are likely to find such goals unacceptable. Use of such screening materials may prevent the significant number of patients in these categories who are suitable for the interdisciplinary approach from receiving appropriate care.

Research and teaching

Despite its overwhelming clinical importance, pain research, until recently, was virtually neglected; advances in diagnosis and therapy have not been commensur-

Table 6–6. Admission criteria for patients with chronic pain

1.	Complete medical and psychiatric evaluation; no overt psychiatric problems; no malingerers or those who have character disorders and have no discernible career goals.
2.	A pain problem of six months or longer
3.	No related malignant disease
4.	No specific medical, surgical, or other psychiatric treatment approach applicable
5.	No litigation. Patients not receiving significant amounts of compensation
6.	Acceptance by the patient of the treatment program
7.	The patient agrees to involve a family member or significant other person in the treatment
8.	Adequate insurance coverage
9.	Absence of ongoing problems with drug addiction.

ate with most other biomedical scientific achievements. Teaching and research are essential to progress but because of service commitments to patients, are usually neglected. Not only is research needed to find new methods of treatment, but there are also needs for epidemiological studies of chronic pain and studies of the relationship of pain treatment to cancer terminal care. To allow pursuit of new knowledge, facilities at major centers for pain treatment need better organization. Perhaps research could be undertaken more effectively on a regional basis.

The multiple, complex issues involved in diagnosis, assessment, and treatment of intractable pain cannot be adequately addressed by the clinical resources of one individual or any one medical discipline. In addition to clinical complexity, sophisticated pharmacological, anatomical, psychological, and technological research must be harnessed, collated, and, where appropriate, subjected to clinical trial. It is a daunting prospect to provide satisfactory service while addressing research in a university teaching hospital, let alone a small community hospital, or even worse, on a personal basis.

Other problems for pain clinic personnel include the burden of data collection on professional and technical staff, the cost effectiveness of data systems, validity and reliability of measurement, excessive or irrelevant data in the system, and behavioral obstacles to new systems and their effective use. Frequently, a data base designed for patient care has no utility for institutional management and policy formulation because of differences in content, level of detail, and timing. Multilevel information systems that can be expanded or contracted in detail and are designed to provide data of established utility are clearly needed in rehabilitation.

Whether early efforts to establish a pain center reflect a clinical or research emphasis, they should be linked as soon as possible. In most instances it is possible to start clinical research soon after establishment of the center without additional funding if the format for a patient data base to be collected and stored is agreed upon. As research meetings must continue, a coherent program must be developed, documented, and periodically evaluated and updated.

With time, a multifaceted program of greatly expanded research and research training programs can be formed and highly effective teaching programs for students and practitioners developed. Other branches of medicine, the public, Congress, federal, state, and municipal governments, insurance carriers, scientific writers, and many others must be informed so they will understand the magnitude of the human and economic impact of pain.

A survey to learn how pain control is taught in anesthesiology residencies indicates that almost half of the these residencies in the United States have no allotted time devoted to teaching residents pain control.[64] Pain education is still conducted within specialties, and each discipline trains residents and fellows to "do their thing" as it has been done in the past. Thus, neurosurgeons treating pain continue to cut nerve tracts, anesthesiologists needle patients, and orthopedic specialists do reconstructive procedures. Needed is an integrated, interdisciplinary training program using trained personnel. Each speciality must accept responsibility for assessing and organizing the roles of its physicians who participate in pain control. This has important implications for training programs, which need to be modified appropriately to meet the new challenge.

Trainees specializing in pain management should be allowed sufficient time to acquire knowledge in pain syndromes. It is important to deemphasize their role as technicians interrrupting nerve pathways and emphasize their role as clinicians seeking to improve a patient's welfare. The trainee will need to make informed referrals to specialists and develop skill in integrating acquired techniques into a total patient management plan. Their roles as educators of other physicians must be expanded so that referrals to pain clinics are made early and narcotic addiction and negative behavior patterns do not develop. Finally, their skills in techniques and medication management must be integrated into a comprehensive pain program directed toward simultaneous management of several aspects of the patient's experience and/or complete rehabilitation.

Currently, much effort is directed toward a national program of public information and teaching and training of physicians to discourage unprofessional operations. At the same time, the Commission on Accreditation of Rehabilitation Facilities (CARF), in collaboration with the American Pain Society, has emerged as the accrediting agency for pain control facilities and development of the concept of the "algology team." The American Academy of Algology is supporting the formation of an American Board of Algology to maintain high academic standards of excellence in the practice of algology.

Communication

Unfortunately, despite advances in the management of chronic pain, very little information is available in the medical literature for a novice in the field to develop a comprehensive pain center in a university hospital. Education of pain clinic staff may suffer because of heavy service commitments. Frequently, the community at large, including the medical community, may not be aware of the existence and function of pain clinics.

In addition to self-education and daily or weekly interdisciplinary patient pain presentation, the following mechanisms may also enhance education of the pain clinic staff: a weekly research meeting, a weekly newsletter, formal or informal communication with community physicians, patient education classes, a public awareness program, and wellness behavior education.

A weekly communication document should be sent to consultants, involved department chairpersons, and other key individuals. The document, which relates the schedule for conferences and program development issue and may occasionally describe a philosophical position for discussion, can maintain communication between the consultants.

Hospitals and medical centers should make every attempt to circulate to community physicians letters describing services offered by their pain center. Hospital annual reports are another valuable tool for communicating with sources of funding such as members of the general assembly and board of trustees. A report from hospital administration that focuses on major undeveloped areas in the delivery of ambulatory care should include the developing pain clinic.

Physician education in the community can be enhanced by offering a three-month miniresidency program to community physicians. Lectures, workshops, and specific courses also should be made available for training inhospital residents and faculty members who do not participate directly in the pain center activities.

Patient care can be further improved by offering patient education, monthly sessions for large groups of patients, and daytime sessions for small groups. A bulletin or newsletter containing patient education information can be disseminated in communities throughout the center's service area.

REHABILITATION OF PATIENTS WITH CHRONIC PAIN

Current role of pain centers

Pain clinics are still in their infancy when it comes to rehabilitation. Today, a very few select pain centers offer rehabilitation programs for patients with chronic pain. The comprehensive rehabilitation approach is aimed at teaching the patient to self-regulate key psychophysiological events contributing to pain. This teaching is augmented by intense physical programs that can lead to total vocational rehabilitation and a more normal lifestyle.

There is little recognition by third-party payers and hospital funding agencies of what constitutes adequate rehabilitation services by pain clinics. Long-term program evaluation presents numerous problems. It is costly in both time and resources. Data are difficult to assemble and often incomplete. Progress between discharge and follow-up is difficult, if not impossible, to assess. Comparative studies in the field require agreement for criteria of success. We have proposed steps in the development of such criteria (see table 6–7).

In rehabilitation of pain patients, primary prevention involves measures to avoid the occurence or onset of chronic pain. Secondary prevention involves early detection and treatment of chronic pain. Tertiary prevention attempts to minimize the present residual effect (impairment, disability, or handicap) and future consequences of chronic pain through monitoring and remediation, that is rehabilitation.

Currently, many components of the health care system are involved with tertiary prevention. However, in rehabilitation in pain clinics, the timing, duration, and use of an interdisciplinary team create multiple opportunities for primary and secondary prevention. Furthermore, the rehabilitation process gradually unfolds over a substantially longer period than does the acute problem. This provides extended opportunities for members of the pain rehabilitation team to become familiar with their patients, to assess their lifestyles, to determine their physical and emotional responses to their illness or injury, to determine factors placing patients at risk for additional adverse outcomes, and to assess risks that are potentially correctable. Unfortunately, many pain clinics do not use these opportunities to full potential. For example, a pain rehabilitation team, by definition, is not involved in crisis management. Unlike the acute care team that provides care for a patient following a traumaic event, they may not participate in primary rehabilitation but may first encounter the patient after tertiary rehabilitation has failed.

Future challenges

Early intervention and prevention programs have the highest potential for reinforcing pain-free behavior before the pain behavior has been learned. Incorporating prevention integrated with acute care into rehabilitation services could lead to a highly efficient health management strategy, providing patients with long-term health benefits and expending the concept and role of rehabilitation facilities.[65] Effective rehabilitation based on prevention is beneficial to the patient, rehabilitation facility, and health policy. Such a rehabilitation program is in a good position to evaluate the population of acute pain patients who are progressing toward chronic pain status. Through prevention, the pain treatment team may reduce the economic impact of chronic pain on society.

Cost of program and alternatives

At present the cost of an inpatient pain program or rehabilitation program is staggering. However, these costs are miniscule compared to the costs of continuing chronic pain, suffering, and disability when patients do not receive adequate pain therapy. With clinical experience, it is hoped that more efficient and less expensive hybrid treatment methods will be developed. The pain centers at the University of North Carolina and the University of Virginia have already demonstrated that outpatient models get results comparable to those of inpatient care at far less costs in time and money to both the patient and society.

Shifting some of the burden of rehabilitation away from the interdisciplinary centers to other medical areas run by family physcians and commnunity pain clinics may be an effective intervention at early levels of pain experience. This will be discussed later under the heading of The Role of Primary Care Physicians.

Currently, various states are becoming incresingly dependent on for-profit companies for ownership and management of its hospitals. In the United States, almost all for-profit hospitals are owned by large national corporations. This national trend towards for-profit involvement is so strong that many hospital management experts believe it will continue. In the future, community hospitals will eventually be faced with a decision to join or sell to a multi-institutional arrangement. Commercial franchising of pain clinics may become commonplace if large national corporations buy freestanding pain clinics, run them from a central office, and employ physicians.

Other changes in the health care industry may also impact on the development of pain clinics. Many speciality and ambulatory surgery clinics are popping up around the country. With the advent of such clinics, patients will not be expected to stay in the hospital after surgery. Insurance companies are forcing new economies on the health care field, and county commissioners are reluctant to spend tax money on capital improvements and indigent care. Insurance companies and Medicare will not continue to tolerate exorbitant charges from inpatient approaches. They will put a cap on their total reimbursement for any pain problem per year. Pain clinics run by for-profit companies may have a better chance of survival in this climate. Only time will tell if the growth of the for-profit hospital industry is a Godsend or a deterrent to the development of pain clinics.

EVALUATION OF DISABILITY

Generally speaking, disability refers to the incapacity of the individual to meet certain standards of physical efficiency and/or social, occupational, or economic responsibility.[66] The current system for evaluating disability in patients with chronic pain is complex, unsophisticated, insufficient, unfair, expensive, chaotic, and in dire need of reassessment.[67] Pain programs, although in an ideal position to address the disability of chronic pain patients, did not actively participate in CARF until recently when pressured by state and federal agencies to participate after obtaining a mandatory accreditation.

Return to work is a highly regarded indicator of total rehabilitation. Yet even the best rehabilitation facilities, such as Rosomoff's is Miami [68] and Seres' in Portland[69], report that fewer than 25 percent of their most successful cases are working two years after treatment. Many patients are so well entrenched in the chronic pain cycle when they are referred that progress is likely to be minimal because the positive rewards for pain behavior have become too firmly established. The best rehabilitation programs feel that people in pain quit work when continuous labor has become difficult. Once they have lost the work habit, they are likely to return only when they feel capable, not when they are no longer disabled.

Medicine and psychiatry have a responsibility to recognize the problem of the growing trend toward chronic disability. These physician specialists must view this problem with alarm, but they themselves should not be "totally and permanently disabled" by the situation.[66] One must realize that there are no clear answers to these difficult issues but only some suggested solutions. They must educate their medical colleagues that social policies shape illness behavior, and that to understand disability, they must understand the disease process and psychological needs of the patients. These doctrines should also be introduced into the medical curricula.

Pain managers in interdisciplinary pain centers must give scientific orientation to the issue of disability. Research must be carried out to study etiology, pain mechanics, standard ways to assess disability, and predictions of treatment outcome. Ways to optimize functioning in patients with chronic pain must be designed. The pain program must include industrial psychologists, lawyers, priests, financial managers, and other nonmedical experts to help on issues related to societal, political, cultural, and economic forces. Pain managers, by educating patients, referring physicians, and congressman about how the disability process reinforces illness behavior, can help cut down the bureaucracy involved with disability compensation.

Many models have been proposed; for example, the New Zealand system of no-fault accident compensation is considered ideal by some.[70–71] To control costs, a national extension of the Florida system, whereby the only facilities approved for rehabilitation are those approved by CARF may be a valid approach. Unfortunately, this organizaton emphasizes facilities rather than quality of program or personnel. Another alternative is to see that the governmental departments of education accredit facilities.

THE ROLE OF PRIMARY CARE PHYSICANS

The family physician has the major task of establishing a diagnosis and commencing treatment for all patients who complain of pain. Not every patient with complex chronic pain is referred to an interdisciplinary pain center. Often the primary care physician is called upon to provide relief. Should the pain become chronic or the condition life-threatening, the family physician may feel obligated to supervise long-term treatment and offer appropriate adivce and support to both patients and family. Such continuing care by the family physician is the cornerstone of patients in the terminal stages of cancer, when pain is commonly a prominent symptom.[72]

Over the last 20 years, however, family physicians have not kept up with advancements in the mangement of chronic pain. The primary care internist/family physician often receives limited training in the behavioral aspects of medicine and, as a result, is less able to obtain and apply the knowledge and skills necessary to effectively help the patient handle the mutually interacting somatic, psychological, and sociological dimensions of chronic pain. Patients with chronic pain usually require a great deal of time and effort for proper management, more time than some physicians may be willing to spend. Also, medical education increasingly tends to neglect family physician training in favor of increasing subspecialization, training that sometimes produces coldly impersonal physicians lacking "samaritanism." Many newly trained physicians have a tremendous desire to learn new medical technology but have a very poor tolerance for patients with chronic pain. Frequently, family physicians treat chronic pain as an emergency and pressure the pain clinic to admit patients if the administration of one or two analgesics is not therapeutic. In addition to poor training in pain management, family physicians are further influenced by pain managers who treat chronic pain as if it were a mystery and perpetuate the myth that the interdisciplinary pain clinic approach is the only way to treat chronic pain, thus discouraging participation of the family physician.

Although the interdisciplinary approach is usually followed by specially equipped pain centers, it is possible to implement a similar treatment strategy in general office practice, and to use some of the techniques discussed without having to refer the patient. Family physicians, by showing interest in pain patients and by keeping in close touch with members of the pain team, can learn the basic principles of chronic pain management. Occasionally attending an interdisciplinary pain conference on their patients or watching videotaped sessions of the conference may enhance family physicians' knowledge. As in any new field of medicine, self-education is also an importance factor in chronic pain management.

Family physicians participate in the management of chronic pain patients in many different way.[73] Once the factors responsible for propagation of the chronic pain syndrome are understood and recognized, the referring doctor can become the primary investigator of treatment to prevent the pain from becoming chronic. Furthermore, adequate relief of acute pain, support during the domestic crisis, pharmacological control of depression or anxiety, referral to relevant social services, avoidance of addictive or sedative "on-demand" drugs, and psychological support are all within the realm of the general practitioner and will reduce the subsequent misery of a substantial number of patitents. Patients should be referred to a pain clinic when the family physician realizes that pain is becoming refractory to simple methods, when personality traits or psychological factors are predominant, or when the greater range of specialist treatment modalities is likely to be beneficial.

Chronic pain is becoming less mysterious. There is hope that, with increasing knowledge and understanding, the chronic pain syndrome will be widely treated without undue difficulty or continuing frustration. Family physicians will be able to prevent pain from becoming chronic and to treat the chronic sufferer when needed. They can also make informed referral to a pain clinic when necessary. Most importantly, they can maintain continuity of care and support despite initially poor therapeutic outcome. Their role can enhance the successful management of the pain patient.

In the last couple of decades, America's romance with medicine has begun to sour. Doctors are no longer placed on a pedestal, nor is medical technology revered as it once was. Medical costs, malpractice insurance, and health care delivery expenses have soared. The greatest imperative need is to place the interdisciplinary approach of the pain clinic in a context that does not exaggerate its social potential and dilute the role of family physicians in the rehabilitation of patients. The team approach in health care and human services is not a new concept.[74–76] Silver[77] used a team approach in primary health centers as early as the late 1940s. Failure to achieve good pain relief from treatment by a primary level physician is an admission of the failure of medical education rather than an argument for the proliferation of pain clinics. Indiscriminate substitution of an interdisciplinary approach for personal care involving the compassion and common sense delivered by the "old time doc" who treated every patient, not just disease, is not only ineffective but also expensive.

MANAGEMENT OF PATIENTS WHO FAIL TO BENEFIT FROM INTERDISCIPLINARY PAIN MANAGEMENT

The group of patients who are not helped by established pain clinicians varies from 14 percent to 56 percent on follow-up.[64] Only a few studies address this group of dissatisfied or problem patients.[68, 69, 70] Little is known about their psychological and behavioral features. Furthermore, there are no reports of treatment programs systematically trying to identify or remediate problem patients.

Most of these unfortunate patients, who are thought to have adaptive limitations characterized by major dependency needs, do not improve despite program participation. These patients often feel dissatisfied because they believe they have organic diseases that are being treated wrongly. They do not improve because their goals are at odds with the program's goals. Some have given up on medicine, and others do not want to return to responsibility. This could be alleviated if the patients are educated and given ample opportunity to review the program as observers.

Another group of patients not helped by the interdisciplinary approach are those who are deleted from admission to pain clinics by very stringent criteria, as discussed earlier. Although a pain clinic may not be the optimum facility for all, these unfortunate patients certainly need understanding and treatment. Experience shows that some patients do not seek further help but learn to live with pain. Others seek further help from other hospitals, medical centers and pain clinics, or community physicians. Many do well with other programs and/or physicians who may employ different attitudes and different management approaches.

CONCLUSIONS

The remarkable growth of interest in and the complexity of pain clinics demand that their present role be critically examined. There is no doubt that real progress has been made in the treatment of intractable pain during the past two decades. The main slogans of the clinical campaign for the last 15 years have been to recognize chronic pain as a separate entity from acute pain and to manage chronic pain by joining an interdisciplinary pain clinic. The campaign has succeeded in raising awareness that medicine and society have overlooked the scientific study of one of their greatest problems. Gradually, we have began to understand the pathophysiology of various chronic pain states.

Unfortunately, the rapid growth has been somewhat disorganized and lacking in direction. The medical profession is burdened with managing an overwhelming number of chronic pain patients, perplexed by many aspects of the pain, confused by many conflicting theories, and inundated with techniques intended to modify the pain. Exploitation of the new field and abuse of the interdisciplinary pain clinic approach are common. Some clinics exists principally to enhance the status and financial security of individuals, departments, or hospitals. Alternatively, some clinics find themselves at risk for becoming a dumping ground for incurables, malingerers, and others for whom pain has become a way of life. Because pain mechanisms have been poorly defined, pain managers continue to treat a variety of chronic pain syndromes under the single generic term *chronic pain*, with prepackaged managements that usually are not effective. The term *interdisciplinary approach* is sometimes used as a gimmick to imply that the pain clinic employs a team of pain experts to solve complex pain problems. Absent are more important ingredients such as specialized, well-integrated programs, personalized care, patient care, family participation, comprehensiveness, continuity of care, and staff dedication.

At this point, fundamental scientific orientation to the issues of acute and chronic pain is needed. To address the scope and magnitude of pain issues, research inquiries and controlled studies must be directed toward the specification of etiologic variables, standardized assessment of physical and psychological characters of subgroups of patients with chronic pain, predictions of treatment outcome, and evaluation of innovative treatment programs designed to optimized functioning subsequent to illness and injury.

Although pain centers succeed in removing some patients' problems or symptoms, a majority of patients must cope with life and its attendent problems in the face of persistent disability. It is for that reason alone that pain clinic programs are urged to broaden their treatment goals, consider more eclectic treatment approaches, and not be satisfied with narrow measures of treatment outcome.

Timely, available, accessible services and personal and family assistance can foster the adaptive coping responses needed to offset a broad range of physiological and anatomical impairments, psychological disturbances, and physical, social, vocational, economic, and architectural barriers to activity and self-realization.[79] The purposes of rehabilitation are applicable to many persons who are believed "noncurable" in the traditional medical sense. Component rehabilitation services are necessary to support and maintain the best possible health status for most persons receiving long-term care.

To achieve the task, training of algologists and family physicians to provide continuity of care may be necessary. The problem of suffering must be directly addressed in medical education. In addition to their service requirements, interdisciplinary pain clinics must participate in physicians' education and training in chronic pain management and in basic and clinical research on pain. Health professionals must educate themselves and receive training in an interdisciplinary pain clinic, if possible. Only through well-organized programs and training of health professionals can we prevent exploitaton and abuse of the interdisciplinary approach. To eradicate chronic pain, it may become necessary to implement a long-range plan to change societal and medical attitudes toward pain and disability.

The interdisciplinary approach to chronic pain offers an alternative to the traditional medical/surgical approach in that it addresses suffering as well as pain. Teamwork and coordination are likely to become more important in the future to avoid fragmentation of medical services from the current trend of increasing specialization. The interdisciplinary approach is here to stay and will continue to flourish in many university hospitals, but its role needs to be redefined. Most of the studies supporting the effectiveness of the approach deal only with the well-being of a small group of select patients. Few studies address problems of managing a large number of patients in a cost-effective manner and maintaining the satisfaction of the participating clinicians. We must control cost, yet expand service. We must search for new therapeutic modalities and develop indices to measure the effectiveness of the program. We must realize that the best way to deal with chronic pain is to prevent an acute problem from becoming progressive and chronic. With continued experience, modeling, and remodeling of the program, it is believed that this approach will achieve a high index of success with rehabilitation and full activity as the ultimate obligatory goal.

REFERENCES

1. Arakawa K: Outpatient pain clinic: review of a two-year experience. J Kans Med Soc 82:292–294, 1981.
2. Devoghel JC: A pain clinic: the fiirst thousand cases. Acta Anesth Belgica 31:197–202, 1980.
3. Swerdlow M: The pain clinic. Brit J Clin Prac 26:403–407, 1972.
4. Wang JK, Ilstrup DM, Nauss LA, Nelson DO, Wilson PR: Outpatient pain clinic: a long-term follow up study. Minn Med 63:663–666, 1980.
5. Bonica JJ: Preface. New approaches to treatment of chronic pain: a review of multidisciplinary pain clinics and pain centers. NIDA Research Monograph Series 36, DHHS Pub No (ADM) 81–1089. Edited by Ng LKY. Washington, D.C.: Department of Health and Hieman Services, May 1981, pp VII–X.
6. Swerdlow M: Four years' pain clinic experience. Anaesthesia 22:568–574, 1967.
7. Gregg JM, Ghia JN: Comparative aspects of chronic pain in the head and neck versus trunk and appendages: experiences of the multidisciplinary, University of North Carolina Pain Clinic. New approaches to treatment of chronic pain: a review of multidisciplinary pain clinics and pain centers. NIDA Research Monography Series 36, DHHS Pub No (ADM) 81–1089. Edited by Ng LKY. Washington, D.C.: Department of Health and Human Services, May 1981, pp 112–117.
8. Ghia JN, Gregg JM: The University of North Carolina Pain Center. I. Organization and function. Anesth Pro 29:41–46, 1982.
9. Ghia JN: The organization of a pain center. J Ambul Care Manage 6:66–77, 1983.
10. Ghia JN, Sugioka K: Are pain centers viable? NCMJ 43:493–495, 1982.
11. International Association for the Study of Pain. Pain terms: a list of definitions and notes on usage. Pain 6:249–252, 1979.
12. Bonica JJ: Introduction to narcotic analgesics in the treatment of cancer and postoperative pain. Acta Anesth Scand (suppl 74) 26:5–10, 1982.
13. Bonica JJ: Important clinical aspects of acute and chronic pain. In: Beers RF Jr, Bassett EG (eds) Mechanisms of Pain and Analgesic Compounds. New York: Raven Press, 1979, pp 15–29.
14. Foley KM: Assessment of pain. Clin Oncol 3:17–31, 1984.
15. Dehen H, Willer JC, Combier J: Congenital indifference in pain and endogenous morphine-like system. In: Bonica JJ, Liebeskind JC, Albe-Fessard DG (eds) Advances in Pain Research and Therapy, vol 3. New York: Raven Press, 1979, pp 553–557.
16. Black RG: The clinical syndrome of chronic pain. In: Ng LKY, Bonica JJ (eds) Pain Discomfort and Humanitarian Care. New York: Elsevier, 1980, pp 207–219.
17. Addison RG: Chronic pain syndrome. Amer J Med 77(3a):54–58, 1984.
18. Pinsky J: Chronic intractable benign pain: a syndrome and its treatment with intensive short-term group psychotherapy. J Human Stress 4:17–21, 1978.
19. Pinsky J: The behavioral consequences of chronic intractable benign pain. Behav Med 5:12–20, 1980.
20. Strang Jp: The chronic disability syndrome. In: Aron off GM (ed) Evaluation and Treatment of Chronic Pain. Baltimore: Urban & Schwarzenberg, 1985, pp 603–623.
21. Fordyce WE: Pain viewed as learned behavior. Adv Neurol 4:415–422, 1974.
22. Fordyce WE: Behavioral Methods for Chronic Pain and Illness. St. Louis: Mosby, 1976.
23. Engel GL: Psychogenic pain and pain-prone patients. Am J Med 26:899–918, 1959.
24. Roy R: Pain clinics: Reassessment of objectives and outcomes. Arch Phys Med Rehab 65:448–451, 1984.
25. Hendler N: Diagnosis and Nonsurgical Management of Chronic Pain. New York: Raven Press, 1981, pp 12–15.
26. Gildenberg PL, DeVaul RA: The Chronic Pain Patient. New York: Karger, 1985, pp 22–40 (Pain and Headache Series. Editor Gildenberg PL, vol 7).
27. Ominsky AJ: Evaluation and treatment of patients with chronic pain. ASA Refresher Courses Anesthesiology 5:137, 1977.
28. Wolff BB: Methods of testing pain mechanisms in normal man. In: Wall PD, Melzack R (eds) Textbook of Pain. Edinburgh: Churchill Livingstone, 1984, pp 186–194.

29. Reading AE: Testing pain mechanisms in persons in pain. In: Wall PD, Melzack R (eds) Textbook of Pain. Edinburgh: Churchill Livingstone, 1984, pp 195–204.
30. Bonica JJ: Local anesthesia and regional blocks. In: Wall PD, Melzack R (es) Textbook of Pain. Edinburgh: Churchill Livingstone, 1984, pp 541–557.
31. Ghia JN, Toomey TC, Mao W, Duncan G, Gregg JM: Toward an understanding of chronic pain mechanisms: the use of psychologic tests and a refined differential spinal block. Anesth 50:20–25, 1979
32. Winnie AP, Ramamurthy S, Durrani A: Diagnostic and therapeutic nerve blocks: recent advances in techniques. In: Bonica JJ (ed) Advances in Neurology. New YorK: Raven Press, 1974, pp 455–460.
33. Marks RM, Sachar EJ: Undertreatment of medical inpatients with narcotic analgesics. Ann Intern Med 78:173–181, 1973.
34. Charap AD: The knowledge, attitude and experience of medical personnel treating pain in the terminally ill. Mt. Sinai J Med (NY) 45:561–580, 1978.
35. Goodwin JS, Goodwin JM, Vogel AV: Knowledge and use of placebos by house officers and nurses. Ann Intern Med 91:106–110, 1979.
36. Bonica JJ: Advances in Neurology, Vol 4. Proceedings of the International Symposium on Pain. New York: Raven Press, 1974.
37. Bonica JJ, Albe-Fessard D: Advances in Pain Research and Therapy, vol I. Proceedings of the Second World Congress on Pain. New York: Raven Press, 1979.
38. Bonica JJ, Liebeskind J, Albe-Fessard D: Advances in Pain Research and Therapy, Vol III. Proceedings of the Second World Congress on Pain. New York: Raven Press, 1979.
39. Bonica JJ, Ventafridda V: Advances in Pain Research and Therapy, Vol II. International Symposium on Pain and Advanced Center. New York: Raven Press, 1979.
40. Ghia JN, Duncan GS, Scott DS, Gregg JM: Therapeutic nerve blocks for chronic pain. Family Medicine 20:74–78, 1979.
41. Ghia JN: The management of chronic pain: an evaluation of recent developments, with special reference to the regional anesthesia and the pain clinic. NCMJ 38:390–392, 1977.
42. Ghia JN: The role of the anesthesiologist in a pain center (with emphasis on the regional anesthesia techniques for pain relief). Reg Anesth 8:166–170, 1983.
43. Huskesson EC: Measurement of pain. Lancet 2:1127–1131, 1974.
44. Berthold WB: Measurement of Human Pain. New York: Raven Press, 1980, pp 173–184.
45. Hanks GW: Depression and anxiety in pain clinic patients, rapid assessment by microcomputer. Anaesthesia, 40:676–679, 1985.
46. Janowsky DS, Sternbach RA: The patient with pain. In: Abram H (ed) Basic Psychiatry for the Primary Care Physician. Boston: Little Brown, 1976, pp 99–116.
47. Egbert LD, Battit GE, Welch CE, Bartlett MK: Reduction of post-operative pain by encouragement and instruction to patients—a study of doctor-patient rapport. Engl J Med 270:825–827, 1964.
48. Mackenzie RS: Psychodynamics of pain. J Oral Med 23:75–84, 1968.
49. Stross JK, Mikkelson WM: Educating patients with osteoarthritis. J Rheumatol 4:313–316, 1977.
50. Parker J, Singsen B, Hewett J, Walker S, Hazelwood S, Hall P, Holston D, Rodon C: Educating patients with rheumatoid arthritis: a prospective analysis. Arch Phys Med Rehab 65:771–774, 1984.
51. Ng LKY: New approaches to treatment of chronic pain: a review of multidisciplinary pain clinics and pain centers. NIDA Research Monograph Series 36, DHHS Pub No (ADM) 81-1089. Washington, D.C.: Department of Health and Human Services, May 1981.
52. Aronoff GM, Evan WO, Enders PL: A review of follow-up studies of multidisciplinary pain units. Pain 16:1–11, 1983.
53. Howland DE, Howland LE: An outpatient pain service. Contemp Anesth Pract 1:55–70, 1978.
54. Moya F: Treatment of osteoarthritis of the spine and herpetic neuralgia at the pain center, Mount Sinai Medical Center. New approaches to treatment of chronic pain: a review of multidisciplinary pain clinics and pain centers. NIDA Research Monograph Series 36, DHHS Pub No (ADM) 81-1089. Edited by Ng LKY. Washington, D.C.: Department of Health and Human Services, May 1981, pp 118–121.
55. Cairns D, Thomas L, Mooney V, Pace JB: A comprehensive treatment approach to chronic low back pain. Pain 2:301–309, 1976.
56. Roberts AH, Reinhardt L: The behavioral management of chronic pain: long-term follow-up with comparison groups. Pain 8:151–162, 1980.

57. Gerschman JA, Burrows GD: Orofacial pain. Aust Fam Phys 6:1219–1225, 1977.
58. Gerschmen JA, Burrows GD, Reck PC: Chronic orofacial pain. In: Bonica JJ, Liebeskind J, Albe-Fessard D (eds) Advances in Pain Research and Therapy, vol 3. New York: Raven Press, 1979, pp 317–322.
59. Kremer EF, Block A, Gaylor MS: Behavioral approaches to treatment of chronic pain: the inaccuracy of patient self-report measures. Acta Phys Med Rehab 62:188–191, 1981.
60. Painter JR, Seres JL, Newman RI: Assessing benefits of pain center: why some patients regress. Pain 8:101–113, 1980.
61. Maruta T, Swanson DW, Swenson WM: Chronic pain: which patients may pain-management program help. Pain 7:321–329, 1979.
62. Seres NA: The MMPI as a predictive instrument for success of treatment of patients with low back pain in a multidisciplinary treatment center. Master's Thesis. University of Oregon Health Sciences Center, Portland, 1976.
63. Swanson DW, Swenson WM, Maruta T, McPhee M: Program for managing chronic pain. I. Program description and characteristics of patients. Mayo Clinic Proc 51:401–408, 1976.
64. Spielman FJ, Ghia JN: Pain control teaching in anesthesia pain. Reg Anesth 8:154–157, 1983.
65. Devellis RF, Sauter SVH: Commentary: recognizing the challenges of prevention in rehabilitation. Arch Phys Med Rehabil 66:52–54, 1985.
66. Ludwig AM: The disabled society. Am J Psychoth 35:5–15, 1981.
67. Ziporyn P: Disability evaluation: a fledging science. JAMA 250:873, 1983.
68. Rosomoff HL, Green C, Silbret M, Stelle R: Pain and low back rehabilitation program at the University of Miami School of Medicine. New approaches to treatment of chronic pain: a review of multidisciplinary pain clinics and pain centers. NIDA Research Monograph Series 36, DHHS Pub No (ADM) 81-1089. Edited by Ng LKY. Washington, D.C.: Department of Health and Human Services, May 1981, pp 92–111.
69. Seres J, Painter JR, Newman RI: Multidisciplinary treatment of chronic pain at the Northwest Pain Center. New approaches to treatment of chronic pain: a review of multidisciplinary pain clinics and pain centers. NIDA Research Monograph Series 36, DHHS Pub No (ADM) 81-1089. Edited by Ng LKY. Washington, D.C.: Department of Health and Human Services, May 1981, pp 41–65.
70. Smith R: The world's best system of compensation injury. Brit Med J 284:1243–1245, 1982.
71. Smith R: Problems with a no-fault system of accident compensation. Brit Med J 284:1323–1325, 1982.
72. Dwyer BE: Record trends in pain clinics. Anesthesia and Intensive Care 11:54–55, 1983.
73. Little TF: Chronic pain modern concepts in management. American Family Physician 10:265–270, 1981.
74. Ducanis AJ, Golin AK: The Interdisciplinary Health Care Team. Germantown, Md: Aspen Systems Corp., 1979.
75. Cunningham RM Jr.: The Holistic Health Centers. A New Direction in Health Care. Battle Creek, Mich.: Kellogg Foundation, 1977.
76. Peterson WM, Tubesing DA, Tubesing NL: Holistic health Care: The Process of Engagement. Hinsdale, Ill.: Society of Wholistic Medicine, 1976.
77. Silver GA: Family Medical Care: A Design for Health Maintenance. Cambridge, Mass.: Ballinger, 1974.
78. Swanson DW, Swenson WM, Maruta T, Floreen AC: The dissatisfied patient with chronic pain. Pain 4:367–378, 1978.
79. Spencer WA. The database for rehabilitation services. Medical Care 14:5, (supp): 33–45, 1976.

7. THE STATE OF PAIN IN THE UNITED STATES: PAST, PRESENT, AND FUTURE

STEVEN F. BRENA AND DENNIS C. TURK

Most of the achievements of mankind have evolved through various stages repeated in similar ways, if under different names, on the stage of history and of time: (1) discovery, (2) pioneering, (3) controversy and early development, (4) organization, and (5) accountability. The same process can be easily detected in the evolution of thoughts, conceptualizations, treatments, and management programs for patients with chronic pain. In this chapter, the five stages of development will be reviewed.

THE AGE OF DISCOVERY

For centuries pain was accepted as an existential experience, associated with the process of living and aging. Actually, the experience of pain was often given a transcendental value, as one way to atone the sufferer for his transgressions against physical or spiritual laws. The very root of the word *pain* is derived from the sanskrit root *PU*, meaning "sacrifices," from which the Latin word *poena*, meaning "punishment," originated; both roots have a clear religious significance.[8]

The relationship between pain and states of health was first established in the mid-19th century, when physiology emerged as an experimental science. The age of discovery was characterized by the idea that pain is a specific sensation with its own sensory apparatus. This idea led to the belief that control of pain is possible by acting upon sensory pathways and organs through surgery, nerve blocking, or pharmacological agents. The first part of the 20th century has witnessed a large number of reports about neurosurgical procedures, nerve blocking techniques, and the use of potent analgesic preparations for pain relief. Recently Bonica[5] extensively reviewed the literature peculiar to the age of discovery in pain therapy.

THE AGE OF PIONEERING

The beginning of the age of pioneering can probably be traced to the publication of the monumental book *Management of Pain* by John J. Bonica and the early efforts of other pioneers, including Alexander, Livingston, and Haugen.[5] These pioneers attempted to apply current pain therapies within the conceptual model of "pain clinics" as multidisciplinary units designed to "review difficult diagnostic and therapeutic pain problems ... in a consultant capacity."[6] Most early pain clinics, while attempting to distinguish between acute and chronic pain, still viewed the latter as a temporal extension of a pathological condition within a conventional biomedical model. Most of these clinics used single-modality treatments such as nerve blocks or neurosurgical procedures, depending upon the particular specialty of the medical staff. It is interesting to note that although nerve blocks and surgical procedures for pain control were fairly well accepted, only a few pioneers dared to apply the multidisciplinary concept for management of chronic pain patients within and outside the United States.[6,7,40] The idea of multidisciplinary pain clinics tended to be ignored by most practitioners during the 1950s and 1960s.

During the 1960s a further evolution in the age of pioneering occurred following four important scientific reports. Basmajian[3] demonstrated that motor units in the muscles could be consciously controlled and changes in function could be obtained through learning techniques. Several years later Miller[43] and others demonstrated that autonomic visceral and glandular functioning could also be changed through training and learning. This set the foundation for biofeedback training to modify psychophysiological activity believed to be associated with pain (e.g., muscular hyperarousal). The reports of these authors in the 1960s opened the door for a very prolific age of research in behavioral medicine.

In 1965, Melzack and Wall published their famous article on pain mechanisms in which they proposed the well known gate theory of pain.[42] Their publication provided new insights into the contribution of sensory-discriminative, motivational-affective, and cognitive-evaluative aspects of the experience of pain and triggered an explosion of basic research on the neurophysiology of nociception.

Almost at the same time, Fordyce and his colleagues[30–32] emphasized the role of operant conditioning in problems of chronic pain. According to Fordyce, pain is a subjective phenomenon that can never be observed but is detected in expressions of pain and suffering such as grimacing, moaning, and limping. The "pain behaviors" that communicate pain can be observed and positively reinforced to maintain the behavioral manifestations of pain long after nociceptive stimulation has ceased. Fordyce suggested, therefore, that elimination of reinforcement for pain behaviors coupled with increased reinforcement of "well-behaviors" (e.g., activity) should lead to extinction of the overt manifestation of pain. Fordyce did not imply that the elimination of pain behaviors was synonymous with elimination of pain; rather he suggested that only the objective manifestations would be modified by behavior modification. The subjective experience of pain was not directly addressed by the operant formulation.

More research in the neurophysiology and psychology of pain has been accomplished in the last 15 years than ever before in the history of medicine. These preliminary conceptualizations and the proliferation of research they inspired moved the state of pain to the next stage.

THE AGE OF CONTROVERSY AND EARLY DEVELOPMENT

The foundation of the International Association for the Study of Pain (IASP) in 1974 opened the way for worldwide development of pain control centers.[13, 15] However, a large number of controversial issues were left open to plague the orderly development of pain management programs. We will outline some of these issues.

Acute versus chronic pain

The bulk of neurophysiological research on pain has heavily focused on experimental pain within an acute pain model whereby pain is viewed as the result of nociception and the amount of pain is believed to be directly proportional to the amount of tissue pathology. Such research has improved our knowledge of peripheral nociceptors and pathways that convey nociceptive information to supraspinal areas. However it has left gaps in our understanding of modulation and supraspinal integrative processes. Moreover, the connecting links between experimental, acute, and chronic pain are still largely missing.

Although there is considerable evidence that antinociceptive mechanisms do exist in the spinal cord, the extent to which they account for analgesia is still not clear. It is now established that nociceptive and antinociceptive phenomena are primarily organized to subserve the experience of pain associated with trauma and inflammation. The release of neuropeptides in response to tissue injury seems to result in a generalized pattern of bodily inactivity and emotional hyporesponsiveness to environmental stimuli that appear helpful to biological healing.[27] However, if the pattern is prolonged past the healing stage, inactivity itself may become a source of tonic nociceptive stimulation that, in turn, may evoke patterns of decreased and ever more painful functions in a progressively deteriorating cycle of multiple physiopsychological malfunctions (table 7–1). Research on bodily responses to the state of weightlessness, experienced by astronauts during space flights[44, 45] improved our knowledge on the physiology of inactivity and its likely impact upon states of chronic pain. Indeed, low activity level is one of the most prominent features in many chronic pain patients. Significantly, reports from most multidisciplinary pain control facilities in the United States indicate subjective decrease of pain intensity following psychophysiological reactivation.[2, 46]

Table 7–1. The inactivity syndrome

Body system	Body response
Musculoskeletal system	Activation of patient's trigger points; loss of coordination; osteoporosis, fibrosis, and stiffness of joints.
Cardiovascular system	Activation of the sympathetic system; adrenergic preponderance; increased basal rate; decreased cardiac reserve; dysfunctional anginal pain following efforts in physical activity.
Respiratory system	Decreased strength of respiratory muscles may cause restrictive respiratory impairment.
Digestive system	Decreased gastrointestinal motility and digestive secretion; altered eating habits; constipation; possible malnutrition; obesity.
Urinary system	Hypercalcaemia; urinary retention; urinary tract infection.
Central nervous system	Decreased sensory inputs results in altered sensations; autonomic imbalance may cause poor adaptation in exercise levels; depression; cognitive stagnation and confusion; disordered sleep problems.
Immune system	Decreased secondary immune activity from stress and malnutrition.

*Reprinted with permission from: Brena, S. F., and Chapman, S. L., Acute Versus Chronic Pain States: "The Learned Pain Syndrome." In S. F. Brena and S. L. Chapman (eds.), Clinics in Anaesthesiology. Chronic Pain: Management Principles, London: Saunders, 1985.

Peripheralist–centralist dichotomy

The controversial documentation of the role of peripheral nociception in sustaining chronic pain states has polarized pain specialists into the "peripheralist" or the "centralist" view. Peripheralists consider chronic pain within the pathological model and presumes a direct relationship between stimulation—even if poorly documented—and the ongoing painful experience. They believe that chronic pain can be "fixed" through unimodal interventions, such as nerve blocks, potent analgesic medication, or ablative surgery, intended to suppress peripheral nociceptive activity. Centralists question the presumption of continued peripheral nociception and view most chronic pain states to be of central origin. Presumed central mechanisms of chronic pain would consist of abnormalities in central neuronal circuitry that have been given different names such as sensory epilepsy or sensory "engram" Clinically, the centralists consider most chronic pain states to be of psychological origin, "psychogenic," and believe that they can be "fixed" through proper understanding and treatment of the underlying psychological forces, with no perceived need for peripheral interventions.[25]

Both the unidimensional peripheralist and centralist positions seem inadequate. Rather than viewing pain as peripheral or central, it would seem worthwhile to consider a multidimensional perspective whereby physical factors are integrated with psychological factors.[50,51] Regardless of its etiology, a chronic pain problem that extends over time is likely to impact on all areas of life. Moreover, psychological reactions can lead to maintenance and exacerbation of pain and suffering directly by creating muscle spasm and indirectly by restricting activities. Reduced muscular strength, endurance, and flexibility can in turn produce greater amounts of nociception, incapacity, and disability. This multidimensional perspective might be viewed as a diathesis-stress model. Psychological factors may exacerbate pain in individuals who are predisposed to pain due to weakness associated with prior trauma, disease, or congenital abnormalities. Additionally, environmental sources of positive reinforcement may further serve to maintain pain and suffering. Predisposition to pain may be necessary but insufficient to produce pain in the absence of psychological stress, inadequate coping resources, and operant factors.

Despite ongoing controversy, a consensus among pain specialists presently agrees that many chronic sufferers do fit into the clinical picture of "chronic pain syndrome."[4,26] The Social Security Commission on the Evaluation of Pain[48] has recognized the existence of such a syndrome and has described many of its characteristics, among them inactivity, misusage of drugs, and abuse of the health care system in the absence of identifiable medical or physical findings.

Changing roles of medication for pain

As pain became viewed as learned behavior, drug-taking behaviors were properly identified as "operant" and considered part of a typical "pain behavior."[30] Detoxification programs for patients misusing medication for pain were designed according to principles of contingency management.[31] Elimination of drugs in the regimen of a chronic pain patient was onsidered a crucial step in pain control programs. As accumulating experience from comprehensive pain control facilities was critically analyzed, several factors emerged that changed the role of medication for chronic pain patients.

First, the term *drug addiction* does not appear to apply to the large majority of pain patients. These pain patients do not display compulsive drug-seeking behavior; they take drugs because they have been prescribed by a physician.[26]

Second, drug usage may be useful in selected chronic pain patients, provided that (1) an accurate classification of chronic pain states is provided, (2) the pharmacodynamics of the drugs are properly understood and applied, and (3) drug therapy is combined with the overall goals of pain rehabilitation programs.[10] Twenty years ago the bulk of medication for chronic pain patients consisted of sedatives and minor tranquilizers. Today, these drugs have little place in pain management. Several nonspecific antalgic drugs, prominently the tricyclic antidepressants, have become first-choice drugs in many categories of pain patients. The key point in drug management for chronic pain patients is the individual level of competent coping: Usage and dosage of drugs that enhance these levels are acceptable, with caution, while those that may impair coping skills should be avoided.[9]

Changing role of nerve blocks

For several decades nerve blocks represented the only nonsurgical treatment modality besides drugs for pain control. Recent appreciation of the complex nature of pain has resulted in ongoing controversy about the usefulness of nerve blocking in pain control programs. From a "centralist" point of view, nerve blocks are not only useless but actually psychologically harmful since they may reinforce in the patient the idea that "something is wrong" in the peripheral tissues of the body that could and should be "fixed." The "peripheralist" continues to maintain that repeated nerve blocks may be valuable in interrupting peripheral stimulation to break theoretical "vicious circles of pain."[35] Actually, the same principles underlying correct drug usage in chronic pain patients may be applied to nerve blocks: (1) proper classification of chronic pain states; (2) proper choice of techniques available, chosing first those techniques with the least morbidity risk; and (3) fitting nerve blocks to the overall goals of pain control programs targeted at enhancing patients' competent coping.[12]

Litigation and disability issues

In the early 1970s it was accepted policy for many pain control facilities to refuse treatment for patients with pending legal clams since such claims were considered major noncorrectable, environmental reinforcers for illness behaviors.[30] The few facilities that accepted patients with disability claims and managed them through operant conditioning found that these patients had a higher dropout raté and were less likely to report changes in pain intensity following nerve blocking[18] than comparable patients without disability claims.[33]

Since knowledge of the psychology of pain has evolved, many attitudes toward patients with pending litigation and disability have changed. It is now well established that the litigation-disability process is a very complex problem, where medicolegal, psychosocial, and economic factors play various and often conflicting roles. Brena and Chapman[16,24] have reviewed the issues of pain, disability, and litigation and the social factors impacting them. As information on pain and disability accumulated in the literature, most pain control programs have reversed early policies and are accepting patients with disability claims. However, only a few are willing to provide a structured vocational disability management for such patients.[1,21,47]

Disorganized growth of pain clinics

In 1976 *Medical World News* listed only 17 pain clinics in the entire United States; in 1979 a pain clinic directory published by the American Society of Anesthesiology listed over 285 pain control facilities. A brochure for public information on chronic pain published by the U.S. Department of Health and Human Services in April 1982 (NIH Publication No. 82-2406) estimated that over 800 pain clinics were operating in the United States that year. The American Pain Society and the American Academy of Pain Medicine presently estimate well over 1,000 pain clinics now active in the United States. The growth of pain clinics has responded to real and urgent needs: the waste in human resources and the enormous cost of the chronic pain "epidemic." At least 40 million Americans suffer chronic, recurrent headaches, spend $4 million a year on medications, and lose 65 million workdays a year. About 23 million people have musculoskeletal impairments, a condition that ranks second only to malfunctions of the circulatory system in total cost of treatment and disability payments. Musculoskeletal disorders cost almost $27.5 billion, and were associated with nearly 20 million hospital days, with an average length of stay of about 9 days. Back pain alone accounts for 36 million office visits to physicians in the United States annually.[34]

Unfortunately, some of the mushrooming pain clinics are operated by health professionals with little or no training in the assessment and treatment of pain, algology. Many well-intentioned but unqualified physicians who set up "pain clinics" to broaden the base of their practice are likely to operate such facilities subsidiary to their own specialties rather than as independent, interdisciplinary units. A few unscrupulous individuals may be trying to exploit the need for pain clinics for financial considerations. These adventurers not only harm the future development of pain research and therapy but, worse, they raise false hopes of a "cure" that may lead to attitudes of helplessness among deceived chronic pain patients.

In the early 1980s qualified and concerned professionals mounted a national program of public information, teaching, and training to sustain and expend gains in pain research and management while discouraging unprofessional operations. These activities resulted in events that probably have ended the pioneer stage and laid the groundwork for organization and settlement of the pain control facilities around the world.

THE AGE OF ORGANIZATION

Onset of the age of organization can probably be traced to the year 1983, when the Commission on Accreditation of Rehabilitation Facilities (CARF) included pain control programs in their *Standards Manual for Facilities Serving People with Disabilities* and the American Academy of Pain Medicine was founded.

CARF was incorporated in 1966 in Illinois by the preexisting Association of Rehabilitation Centers and the National Association of Sheltered Workshops and Homebound Programs. CARF and the Joint Commission on Accreditation of Hospitals (JCAH) were associated from 1966 to 1971 when CARF chose to function separately. Several national organizations, among them the American Academy of Pain Medicine, are sponsoring members of CARF. The choice of CARF as the accrediting agency for pain control facilities has been a particularly wise decision, since CARF standards are directed toward multidisciplinary, interdisciplinary facilities with a comprehensive array of modalities directed at a broad collection of clinical syndromes, all of them within the general scope of rehabilitation. Single-disciplinary, modality-oriented, or syndrome-oriented clinics do not usually seek CARF accreditation, since they already are likely to enjoy a full status under the respective departments, especially in large group practices or hospitals. It is conceivable that many such limited pain units may expand to meet the comprehensivity of rehabilitation criteria.

Historically, the American Pain Society led pain facility organization and recommendations for educational and consultative functions. Many of these recommendations later became incorporated in the CARF standards. In 1982 CARF convened 13 regionally distributed, full-time pain center directors to form a National Advisory Committee on chronic pain management programs. Their recommendations were distributed to CARF members and other interested parties, including the American Pain Society Directors. After feedback and adequate consensus, the CARF Board of Directors published the revised recommendations in the CARF Standards Manual. Since the publication of the standards in 1983, 48 pain control programs have been certified, 14 inpatient, 13 outpatient, and 11 both inpatient and outpatient programs (CARF Report, March 1986). State and federal agencies have been slow to require mandatory acceptance of CARF accreditation as a prerequisite for reimbursement of charges for services rendered to chronic pain patients. Presently, the Florida Department of Labor and Employment Security, Division of Workers' Compensation, is the only state agency that mandates CARF accreditation (State of Florida, Chapter No. 38F-8, Rules 38F-8.20 to 38F-8.53).

The American Academy of Pain Medicine was founded with well-defined purposes that are clearly stated in its bylaws: to support the formation of a specialty in algology; to support the formation of an American Board of Algology; to pursue excellence in education as it concerns algology and related sciences; to pursue high standards of excellence in the practice of algology; to uphold high principles, policies, and practices for the attainment of the best in care for the patient suffering with pain; to provide communication with other groups; to preserve and to achieve the principles and purposes of the academy; to develop understanding of the social economic impact of pain and its treatment, in order to develop better approaches to pain patient care and cost containment.

The algology team

The CARF Standards for Pain Control Programs stress the role of the algology team as an interdisciplinary body of health professionals who share a common language and a common philosophy, agree on the same therapeutic goals for each patient, have easy interdisciplinary communication and access to patients' records, and share space for offices and treatment rooms. Members of the algology team play different but equally important roles that are well defined and accepted by consensus in interdisciplinary pain control centers. Crucial members of an algology team include physicians, psychologists, physical and occupational therapists, nurses, and vocational evaluators. Well-accepted roles of the team are to activate, motivate, and educate chronic pain patients so that their lifestyles may be normalized and their dependency on the health care system decreased or eliminated. In this conceptual framework, patients are no longer viewed as "recipients" of therapeutic interventions but rather are trained to become directly involved in their own care and self-maintenance of health.[15]

AGE OF ACCOUNTABILITY—SOME CHALLENGES FOR THE FUTURE

Although the organization process is still in full progress, pain facilities in the United States are already faced with serious challenges. A successful response will ultimately determine the survival of the infant science of algology and the viability of interdisciplinary pain treatment centers. We have entered the age of accountability, which raises a number of challenges for the future.

Multiaxial assessment of pain (MAP)

To establish credibly that pain control facilities are viable alternatives to conventional medicine the key is demonstration of utility. An essential first step is the construction of a multiaxial system for weighted scoring of medical, psychosocial, and behavioral information to document the progress of treatment. This MAP system should be simple and require minimal added effort from health care professionals. Such a system should bring consistency and validity to an otherwise chaotic patient evaluation process.[53,54] To develop a MAP, a valid and reliable assessment battery should accumulate normative information. When norms become available, they can be used to screen chronic pain patients to design treatment modalities and management plans, to predict outcome of treatment, and to provide data necessary for research and comparison of patients across health care facilities. Periodic reevaluation can document patient progress and the successful treatment provided by the pain center.

Perhaps the earliest attempt to evaluate multidimensional factors in pain perception was Melzack's[41] development and description of the McGill Pain Questionnaire. This inventory was designed to assess sensory as well as psychological components of pain. Another early attempt, proposed by Brena and Koch[20] was the Emory Pain Estimate Model (EPEM) for quantification and classification of pain states.

The EPEM is an operational definition of chronic pain patients obtained through the quantification of three sets of data—medical findings, behavioral data, and the relationship between medical-behavioral correlates—expressed in four different classes of chronic pain patients. Brena and Chapman[16,17] have described the clinical characteristics of these four classes of chronic pain patients, their impairment and disability, and the relationship between the classes and

Table 7–2. Multiaxial assessment of pain

Axis I:	*Medical-physical quantification of:* 1. Laboratory and other diagnostic procedures 2. Physical examination
Axis II:	*Psychosocial including patients' perceptions of:* 1. Pain 2. Affective distress 3. Interference of pain with domains of life (e.g., social, vocational, marital, recreational, physical) 4. Responses of significant others
Axis III:	*Behavioral-functional including:* 1. Observable communications of pain and distress 2. Pain-related use of health care system 3. Medication 4. Activity levels 5. Functional mobility, strength, and flexibility

Table 7–3. Average rank-ordering of 18 common medical-physical procedures used in pain assessment

1. Neurological examination
2. Observation of gait and posture
3. Examination of muscular function (tone, mass, strength)
4. Assessment of spinal mobility
5. Examination of soft tissues
6. Assessment of mobility of weight-bearing joints
7. Plain radiography
8. Assessment of mobility of joints other than spine or weight-bearing
9. CT scan
10. Electromyography
11. Contrast radiography
12. Examination of internal organs (inspection, palpation, auscultation, percussion)
13. Nuclear medicine
14. Laboratory tests (other than blood count)
15. Thermography
16. Blood count
17. Electroencephalography
18. Electrocardiography

patient response to nerve blocks for low back pain.[12, 19, 23] Waddell and his colleagues[57] have employed a similar approach although they have focused only on low back pain. The main weakness of EPEM is that its medical and behavioral scoring systems lack the necessary biometric rigor for wide use in scientific research.[53]

Recently, the pain team at the University of Pittsburgh has undertaken the task of developing an acceptable and psychometrically sound system for the quantification and integration of medical-physical, psychosocial, and behavioral-functional data for use with diverse groups of chronic pain patients. Several studies have already been conducted although additional research is needed. Table 7–2 summarizes the components of a comprehensive MAP system.

Axis I of a MAP system should assess medical and physical findings. Quantification of physiological and diagnostic data is essential, yet to date no procedures are available that meet each of four important criteria, namely, (1) psychometrically sound, (2) brief and easy to use, (3) general enough to employ across pain syndromes, and (4) specific to pain including norms for pain patients.

As a first step in the development of a scoring approach that meets these criteria, a survey was conducted to establish the differential utility of the most commonly employed diagnostic procedures used by algologists.[55] Eighty members of the American Academy of Algology were surveyed to establish the differential utility of 18 frequently used diagnostic tests and examination procedures (e.g., electromyography, spinal mobility). The average individual rank-ordering of these procedures, from 1, most useful, to 18, least useful, in the evaluation of pain patients is presented in table 7–3. The physicians sampled displayed a high degree of agreement regarding the relative importance and usefulness of the different procedures included in the survey. The average individual rank-order correlation within this group was .75. If these procedures can be shown to be reliably assessed, the results will be useful in developing a weighted scoring procedure for quantifying medical-physical findings.

Another study was conducted to assess interrater reliability when the survey described above was used to evaluate medical-physical findings. Two algologists at the Pain Control and Rehabilitation Institute of Georgia performed chart reviews of 30 chronic pain patients using 3- or 4-point systems to rate each of the 18 procedures listed in table 7–3. The scoring system included deciding whether a procedure was relevant to the assessment of a specific presenting complaint and, if so, abnormal findings were rated in terms of their severity. Since 16 of the 18 procedures were reliably rated, these preliminary results are promising. In another study in progress two algologists perform physical examinations on the same patients and rate the patient on an instrument refined from the original 18-item survey. Early results seem to predict that a medical-physical findings assessment system that meets the criteria listed earlier can be developed.

Once a satisfactory assessment of axis I, medical-physical data, has been developed, it must be integrated with psychosocial and behavioral-functional data.[50] Procedures for assessing these two additional axes of the Multiaxial Assessment of Pain system are already available and will be described briefly.

Research on chronic pain has been hindered by the unavailability of reliable and valid measures for psychosocial and behavioral-functional contribudors to the suffering of chronic pain patients. Assessments have relied on self-reports of pain intensity and on instruments with no established and acceptable psychometric characteristics. Moreover, assessment inventories have failed to consider substantial evidence in the literature that supports a progression from nociception to autonomic arousal, muscular tension, and dysphoric mood, all of which influence the expression of pain.[28] Moreover, there has been an unfortunate tendency to rely on instruments that were never intended for use with chronic pain patients (e.g., the Minnesota Multiphasic Personality Inventory, MMPI). For some recent cogent comments on this issue see Main.[39]

The West Haven–Yale Multidimensional Pain Inventory (WHYMPI) was developed to enhance the pain assessment armamentarium by including questions that cover a range of life experiences of chronic pain patients.[37] Each of the components of the WHYMPI was based on research suggesting the importance of patients' appraisals, activities, and responses of others to the experience, maintenance, and exacerbation of chronic pain.[30,51] The psychometric evaluation of the WHYMPI demonstrated that it has excellent internal consistency, test-retest reliability, and good convergent and discriminant validity. Moreover, the instrument is brief, less than 60 questions, and easily understood with all questions relevant for people with chronic pain. The inventory is comprised of 12 scales, 8 of which are related to axis II of the MAP system, psychosocial factors. These scales include (1) interference of pain with multiple domains of life (e.g., vocational functioning, social activities), (2) perceived support from significant others, (3) pain severity, (4) perception of control over life and pain problems, (5) negative mood, and three scales related to how patients perceive significant others, responses to their expressions of pain and distress.

A third area particularly important for assessment of chronic pain patients is behavior and function. What are patients doing or failing to do because of their pain and how do they communicate their pain and suffering to others? Axis III, behavioral-functional, can be assessed by the last four scales of the WHYMPI[37] that address performance of specific behaviors (i.e., household chores, outdoor work, social activities, and activities away from home), in conjunction with measures that rate the use of medication and the health care system and with observer ratings of pain behaviors.[30] Several procedures have been developed for the assessment of pain behaviors.[36, 56] A simple 20-item checklist was developed by Turk et al. from surveys completed by pain specialists. Four general areas were identified including (1) distorted ambulation or posture, (2) negative affect, (3) facial/audible expressions of distress, and (4) avoidance of activity.

A comprehensive MAP system should assist in our understanding of chronic pain, facilitate treatment decision making, and serve as a set of criteria for evaluating the efficacy of multidisciplinary pain clinics.

Management of vocational disability

There is a growing awareness at all levels of the U.S. government, labor, management, and the insurance industry that the efficiency and accountability of current systems that evaluate the disability of chronic pain patients need to be improved. This national awareness is expressed in the public law (1980—460, Section 3, Subsection (b), Paragraphs 1–6 of the Social Security Disability Reform Act of 1984) that established a commission to study how chronic pain determines eligibility for disability benefits and to make recommendations about pain evaluation.[48]

There are many systems of disability insurance currently available in the United States. They are administered by the federal government (Social Security Administration, Veterans' Administration), the states (workers' compensation insurance programs), and by the private insurance companies. Although administrative details differ, the majority of disability programs do not award disability benefits on the basis of symptoms alone, including pain, unless medical findings show a pathological condition that could reasonably be expected to produce those symptoms. At the moment there is no recognized system to evaluate pain-related disability, one that would address the issue of work functioning and be acceptable to the various agencies that administer disability programs. According to Ziporyn, misunderstanding and mismanagement of disability cases is rampant, inviting accusations of bias and malpractice.[59]

When assessing disability claims in chronic pain patients, insurance companies, industry, government, legal professionals, and the clients themselves are faced with a chaotic system whereby parties are forced to make judgments from different and often inadequate information. Thus, the claim is often settled in favor of the party who has chosen the better attorney.

The cost of such mismanagement is appalling. For instance, in California the compensation cost in 1972 was $774 million, in 1981 $3 billion. In 1960 employers on the average contributed $346 per worker; in 1978 they contributed $2, 115 per year for benefits for each worker.[47] Pain control facilities in the United States have repeatedly reported that the majority of their referrals have pending disability claims.[3, 16] The claimed disability status is often not matched by clear evidence of a pathological condition and usually has followed a "trivial injury" whose prognostic healing was a few weeks.[58] The private insurance sector and state and federal agencies are increasingly scrutinizing pain control programs to determine if they effectively address the disability issues of chronic pain patients and if they provide meaningful information that may be used to close administrative or legal claims. Patients with a long history of pain and disability claims may be best served by a systematic, comprehensive, functional diagnosis including the following information:

1. Medical-physical, psychosocial, and behavioral-functional data (MAP system).
2. Evaluation of the physical impairment.
3. Evaluation of the residual functional capacity (RFC).
4. Evaluation of the ability to perform vocational tasks within the RFC.
5. Evaluation of the patient's capability to meet actual work duties (work hardening programs) and the feasibility of work adjustments (ergonomics) to keep the worker productive on a long-term basis.

Brena and Spektor[21] have recently described in some detail this structured management program for vocational disability.

Development of algology as a recognized medical specialty

The unique role of the professional algologist is recognized by CARF in its *Standards Manual for Facilities Serving People with Disabilities* (*1986*): "The physician responsible for the person's program should possess training or experience in the management of persons with pain; this should be reflected in the privileges granted by the institution." However, CARF certifies facilities, not individual professionals. At present there is no American Board of Algology; and therefore anybody can claim to be a "pain expert" with minimal training and experience in the field. The establishment of such a board is a long-term goal of the American Academy of Pain Medicine (AAPM), as is clearly stated in its bylaws. Before this goal is obtained, the AAPM is facing another and more basic challenge: to define the specialty of algology itself. At present algology is an impressive Greek name without clear reference to any particular science or discipline. The preliminary survey by Turk et al. cited earlier reveals that there is substantial agreement among algologists concerning the relative importance of specific diagnostic and laboratory procedures in assessment of chronic pain patients.[55] Much more work along these lines is required to identify within the basic sciences the body of common knowledge that will make up the specialty of algology.

Improved management for cancer patients

A major challenge for the future concerns the appropriate treatment of pain among cancer patients. With few outstanding exceptions the bulk of literature describing pain control center operations in the United States focuses upon management of nonmalignant syndromes, mainly back pain and headache. Few centers report clinical and research efforts to manage cancer patients. Yet, many publications have shown that emotional and physical malfunctions are common in cancer patients. Many of these problems, such as altered daily activities, generalized weakness, ambulation difficulties, anxiety and depression, and drug misusage, are likely to respond well to pain control programs since they are similar to disabilities of other etiologies.[22, 29, 38] However, patients with terminal illnesses are too often undermedicated or are victims of drug mismanagement because of wrong choices in drugs, dosages, and administration. Their suffering is increased by anxiety, depression, and adverse drug effects. Correct management of cancer patients is a clear national health challenge that so far has not been met adequately nationwide. Comprehensive long-term management programs for cancer patients should consider three interrelated treatment phases:[52]

Phase 1 (early stage). Oncology therapy plus patient education in self-control of pain through stress management, relaxation techniques, and self-medication, under medical supervision.

Phase 2 (intermediate stage). Continuing oncology supervision plus rehabilitation programs to correct the consequences of heavy oncological intervention and to enhance adequate levels of competent coping.

Phase 3 (terminal illness stage). Discontinued oncology therapy, liberal medication p.r.n. for pain, PO, IM, and IV if necessary. Pain control centers could play important roles during phases 1 and 2 of this long-term comprehensive management program, while hospice programs can provide competent psychosocial support during phase 3.

CLOSING REMARKS

In summary, pain control services in the United States have grown past the pioneer age into the age of accountability. The ultimate challenge for these services is to demonstrate, with scientific rigor, that an algology team can provide alternative approaches to the reliance on unstructured therapy with drugs and surgeries. By applying these approaches to all classes of chronic pain patients, pain control centers may be laying the groundwork of the integration of behavioral medicine and biomedicine that can manage all chronic illnesses. If successful in their responses to the challenges of the future, pain control centers around the world may possibly offer the best health support system for both patients in need of rehabilitation and chronically ill patients.

REFERENCES

1. Aronoff GM: A holistic approach to pain rehabilitation: the Boston Pain Unit. In: Ng, LKY (ed) NIDA Monograph 36. Washington, D.C.: Department of Health and Human Services, 1981.
2. Aronoff GM, Evans WO, Enders PL: A review of follow-up studies of multidisciplinary pain units. Pain 16:1–11, 1983.
3. Basmajian JV: Control and training of individual motor units. Science 141:440–441, 1963.
4. Black RB: The chronic pain syndrome. Surg Clin North Am 55:999–1011, 1975.
5. Bonica JJ: Evolution of pain concepts and pain clinics. In: Brena SF, Chapman SL (eds) Chronic Pain: Management Principles. Clinics in Anesthesiology. London: England: Saunders, 1985.
6. Bonica JJ: Clinical Application of Diagnostic and Therapeutic Nerve Blocks. Springfield, Ill.: Charles C Thomas, 1959.
7. Brena SF: Les cliniques de la douleur. Anesthesiologie Europeene, 230–257, 1961.
8. Brena SF: Pain and Religion. Springfield, Ill. Charles C Thomas, 1972.
9. Brena, SF: Oral analgesic, use and misuse. Emerg Med 23:139–145, 1983.
10. Brena SF: Chronic pain: A structured approach to drug therapy. Mod Med 12:124–144, 1984.
11. Brena SF: Chronic pain states: A model for classification. Psychiatr Ann 14:778–782, 1984.
12. Brena SF: Nerve blocks and chronic pain states: An update, Postgrad 78:62–86, 1985.
13. Brena SF: Pain clinics around the world—an overview. In: Brena SF, Chapman SL (eds) Chronic Pain: Management Principles. Clinics in Anesthesiology. London: Saunders, 1985.
14. Brena SF, Chapman SL: Acute versus chronic pain states: the learned pain syndrome. In: Brena SF, Chapman SL (eds) Clinics in Anaesthesiology. Chronic Pain: Management Principles. London: Saunders, 1985.
15. Brena SF: Pain control facilities: Patterns of operation and problems of organization in the USA. In: Brena SF, Chapman SL (eds) Chronic Pain: Management Principles. Clinics in Anesthesiology. London: Saunders, 1985.
16. Brena SF, Chapman SL: Pain and litigation. In: Wall PD, Melzack, R (eds) Textbook of Pain. Edinburgh: Churchill-Livingstone, 1984.
17. Brena SF, Chapman SL: Chronic pain states and compensable disability: an algorithmic approach. In: Benedetti C et al. (eds) Advances in Pain Research Therapy (vol 7). New York: Raven Press, 1984.
18. Brena, SF, Chapman SL, Bradford LA: Conditioned responses to treatment in chronic pain patients: Effects of compensation for work-related accidents Bull LA neurol Soc 44:48–52, 1979.
19. Brena SF, Chapman SL, et al.: Chronic pain states: Their relationship to impairment and disability. Arch Phys Med Rehab 60:387–389, 1979.
20. Brena SF, Koch DL: The Pain Estimate Model for quantification and classification of chronic pain states. Anesthe Rev 2:8–13, 1975.
21. Brena SF, Spektor S: Disability management of chronic pain patients. In: Warfield CA (ed) The Anesthesiologist's Guide to Pain Management. Hingham, Mass.: Kluwer (in press).
22. Brena SF, Wallace KB: Cancer pain and chronic illness. J Med Assoc Ga 71:55–56, 1982.
23. Chapman SL, Brena SF: Learned helpessness and response to nerve blocks in chronic low back pain patients. Pain 14:355–364, 1982.
24. Chapman SL, Brena SF: Pain and society, Ann Behav Med 7:21–24, 1985.
25. Crue BL: The peripheralist and centralist views of chronic pain. Semin Neurol 3:331–339, 1983.
26. Crue BL, Pinsky JJ: Chronic pain syndrome, four aspects of the problem. In: Ng LKY (ed) NIDA Research Monograph 36, New approaches to the treatment of chronic pain. Washington, D.C.: U.S. Department of Health and Human Services, 1981.
27. Duggan AW: Nociception and anti-nociception in spinal cord. In: Brena SF, Chapman SL (eds) Chronic pain: Management Principles, Clinics in Anesthesiology. London: Saunders, 1985.
28. Flor H, Turk DC, Birbaumer N: Assessment of stress-related psychophysiological reactions in chronic back pain patients. J Consult Clin Psychol 53:354–364, 1985.
29. Foley KM: Current issues in the management of cancer pain: Memorial Sloan Kettering Cancer Center. In: Ng LKY (ed), NIDA Research Monograph 36. Washington, D.C.: Department of Health and Human Services, 1981.
30. Fordyce WE: Pain viewed as learned behavior. In: Bonica JJ (ed) Advances in Neurology (vol 4). New York: Raven Press, 1974.
31. Fordyce WE: Treating chronic pain by contingency management. In: Bonica JJ (ed) Advances in Neurology (vol 4). New York: Raven Press, 1974.
32. Fordyce WE, Fowler RS, DeLateur B: An application of behavior modification techniques to a problem of chronic pain. Behav Res Ther 6:105–107, 1968.

33. Hammonds WH, Brena SF, Unikel IF. Compensation for work-related injuries and rehabilitation of patients with chronic pain. South Med J 71:664—666, 1978.
34. Holbrook TL, Grazier K, et al.: The frequency of occurrence, impact and cost of musculoskeletal conditions in the United States. Paper presented at the annual meeting of the American Academy of Orthopaedic Surgeons, Chicago Illinois, 1984.
35. Katz J: The value of diagnostic and therapeutic nerve blocks: The peripheralist viewpoint. Semin Neurol 3:340–341, 1983.
36. Keefe FJ, Block AR: Development of an observation method for assessing pain behavior in chronic low back pain. Behav Ther 13:363–375, 1982.
37. Kerns RD, Turk DC, Rudy TE: The West Haven-Yale Multidimensional Pain Inventory. Pain 23:345–356, 1985.
38. Lehmann JF. DeLisa JA, et al: Cancer rehabilitation: assessment of need, development, and evaluation of model of care. Arch Phy Med Rehab 59:410–419, 1978.
39. Main CJ: Must we play the MMPI game? (or is the MMPI the only game in town?). In: Broome AK (ed) Readings in Psychology and Pain: Proceedings of the 1st International Conference of the Pain Interest Group. Liverpool: Author, 1984.
40. Maline DB, Crue BL: Evolution of the pain center at the City of Hope Medical Center. In: Crue BL (ed) Pain Research and Treatment. New York: Academic Press, 1975.
41. Melzack, R: The McGill Pain Questionnaire: Major Properties and scoring methods. Pain, 1, 277–299, 1975.
42. Melzack R, Wall PD: Pain mechanisms: a new theory. Science 150:971–979, 1965.
43. Miller NE: Learning of visceral and glandular responses. Science 16:434–445, 1969.
44. NASA SP-368: Biomedical results in Apollo. 1975.
45. NASA SP-377: Biomedical results in Skylab. 1978.
46. Ng, LKY (ed). NIDA Research Monograph 36. New Approaches to Treatment of Chronic Pain. Washington, D.C.: Department of Health and Human Services, 1981.
47. Seres JL, Newman RI: Negative influences of the disability compensation system: perspectives for the clinician. Semin Neurol 3:360–369, 1983.
48. Social Security Administration: Report of Commission on the Evaluation of Pain. Washington, D. C.: Department of Health and Human Services, 1987.
49. Sternbach RA: pain: A Psychophysiological Study. New York: Academic Press, 1968.
50. Turk DC, Kerna RD: Conceptual issues in the assessment of clinical pain. Int J of Psychiatry Med 13:15–26, 1983.
51. Turk DC, Meichenbaum D, Genest M: Pain and Behavioral Medicine: A Cognitive-Behavioral Perspective. New York; Guilford Press, 1983.
52. Turk DC, Rennert KS: Pain and the terminally ill cancer patient. In: Sobel H (ed) Behavior Therapy in Terminal care: A Humanistic Approach. Cambridge, Mass.: Ballinger, 1981.
53. Turk DC, Rudy TE: Assessment of chronic pain states: MAPping out the terrain. J Pain Symp Man (in press).
54. Turk DC, Rudy TE, Boucek CD: The contribution of psychological factors to the experience of chronic pain. In: Warfield CA (ed) The Anesthesiologist's Guide to Pain Management. Hingham Mass.: Kluwer (in press).
55. Turk DC, Rudy TE, Brena SF: Quantification of medical-physical findings in chronic pain. Paper presented at the annual meeting of the American Pain Society, Washington, D.C., 1986.
56. Turk DC, Wack JT, Kerns RD: An empirical examination of the "pain-behavior" construct. J Behav Med 8:119–130, 1985.
57. Waddell G, Main CJ: Assessment of severity in low back disorders. Spine 9:204–208, 1984.
58. Woodyard JE: Injury compensation claims and prognosis. Part II. J Soc Occup Med 30:57–60, 1980.
59. Ziporyn P: Disability evaluation: A fledgling science? JAMA 250:873, 1983.

INDEX